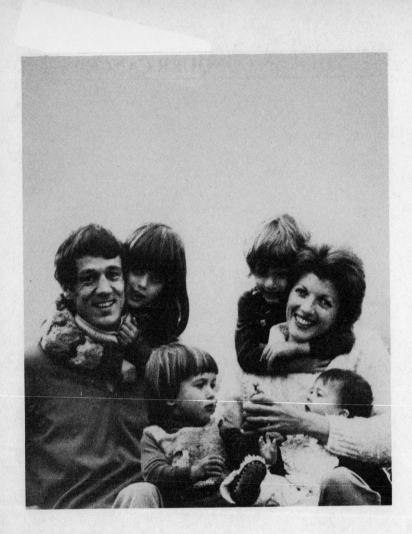

YOU CAN CONQUER CANCER

Ian Gawler

HILL OF CONTENT
Melbourne

By the same Author:
PEACE OF MIND
By Grace Gawler
WOMEN OF SILENCE
The Emotional Healing of Breast Cancer

First published in Australia 1984
by Hill of Content Publishing Company Pty Ltd
86 Bourke Street Melbourne Australia 3000

© Copyright Ian Gawler 1984
12th Reprint

Designed by Josie Semmler
Photography by Derek Hughes
Typeset in 10/12 English Times by Dudley E. King
Printed in Australia by Australian Print Group
Maryborough, Victoria

National Library of Australia
Cataloguing-in-Publication data

Gawler, Ian, 1950–
  You can conquer cancer.

  Bibliography.
  ISBN 0 85572 141 3.
  1. Cancer – Treatment. 2. Therapeutic systems.
  I. Title.

616.99'406

To Grace
– naturally

ACKNOWLEDGEMENTS

In addition to those mentioned in the Introduction, acknowledgement is made to all those authors and publishers of works quoted or cited for reference. These are listed at the end of the book and thereby gratefully acknowledged.

A special note of thanks is due to my fellow veterinarian and typist, Dr Joan Humphreys. Joan is a wonderfully composed, accurate and instructive typist who paused just long enough before the manuscript to use its principles to cure her own rheumatoid arthritis. She also can operate (surgically) quite freely again now.

My thanks also to John Simkin for compiling the index.

Although the case histories in this book are true, the names have been changed to honour the privacy of those concerned. To those and others who may have helped indirectly the author acknowledges his gratitude.

CONTENTS

INTRODUCTION

It's a great feeling to have recovered from cancer – to have been through it all and to be living a full, happy life again. I have done it. I have seen others do it and I know many more will repeat the process in the future. This book, then, is offered with a sense of excitement and joy – the joy in having done it and the excitement of being able to help others do it.

The book examines the patient's role in disease and healing. It is intended as a self-help manual that provides the signposts along the path to total well-being – total health.

Where there's a rhyme there's a reason

My right leg was amputated with *osteogenic sarcoma* (bone cancer) in January 1975. While there were no signs of the cancer anywhere else in my body at that time, only 5 per cent of patients can expect to be alive five years after such surgery. If my cancer reappeared, I was told, it would be expected to be rapidly fatal. Most people die within three to six months of developing secondary growths of this form of bone cancer.

In fact, my cancer did reappear during November of 1975. By March 1976, my specialist thought that I would live for only two more weeks. My subsequent recovery has run the full gamut of available treatments and, in June 1978, I was declared free of active cancer.

Since then my wife Grace and I have had four children, begun a new veterinary practice, taken up a fifteen hectare farm, developed vegetable gardens and orchards and built a new house. In 1981 we initiated the Melbourne Cancer Support Group.

The Support Group grew from an urge to pass on the benefits

of an experience that we believe to be unique. Having been through it all ourselves we understand the problems cancer patients face. Also, being a rather pragmatic veterinarian, I had enough medical knowledge to understand my own position at the outset, evaluate my progress, and assess critically the wide range of treatments considered. Both Grace and I were blessed with open minds, so we were ready to consider anything that worked towards our aim. That aim was to create the right environment in which my body would heal itself. To think that the body can play a major part in healing itself is a novel approach in treating cancer and one which we now know to be full of possibilities.

When my cancer had recurred and the situation looked hopeless from the medical viewpoint, Grace and I remained confident that there *was* another way. Already we had been introduced to the idea that cancer involved a state of immune deficiency. To explain: it is known that throughout the lifetime of every healthy person cancerous cells develop in their body. This is a medically accepted fact. It also is accepted that the body normally recognises these abnormal cells as a potential threat to its health and acts quickly to isolate and destroy them. It does so before any physical symptoms become apparent. However, in cancer patients, this does not happen and the growths continue unopposed. The body offers no resistance and symptoms of cancer are the result.

So we began with the attitude that it was possible to restimulate the body's natural defences – the immune system. This being so, it followed that the body itself could destroy and remove all trace of the cancer. As an extension, if the immune system remained intact and functioning properly, there should be no worry about the cancer reappearing anywhere else. An exciting prospect.

That attitude was our starting point, our basic premise. All we did was directed towards that end. So while we explored so many avenues of treatment, we felt it to be all part of the process of finding the right balance for me. What we are now able to do is recognise the basic ingredients in *our* success and at the same time give our impressions of all the other treatments we tried.

Approached in this light, cancer becomes something of an adventure. It becomes a growing, learning experience. Despite the trials, I am sure both Grace and I have been enriched by all we have been through.

This attitude of adventure, growing and learning through cancer, is so very different to the fears that normally surround the word. Probably no other word strikes as much emotional fear in the community today as does cancer. This fear is based on four basic misconceptions.

The four misconceptions of cancer:
1 The cause of cancer is unknown.
2 Cancer is generally associated with pain and an untimely death.
3 There is nothing patients can do to help themselves except hand over responsibility for their well-being, and indeed their lives, to a doctor.
4 Treatments are unpleasant, and probably will not work anyway.

It is the aim of the Melbourne Cancer Support Group and of this book to dispel these fears, to replace them with a positive attitude and then to show how patients can make a decisive contribution towards restoring their own health.

This book presents the good news on cancer. It is not a book about dying gracefully with cancer. It is about a process of living – living to the full.

The starting point is seeing cancer as a process. We must realize that most of the causes of cancer are now known and that cancer is not a chance happening of random fate. Once the causes are identified it becomes possible to plan appropriate action. To do this satisfactorily we need to expand our horizons. We need to consider the roles of those three aspects of our human condition that we know as *physical, psychological* and *spiritual*.

While I recognise the overriding importance of spiritual factors, I do not confuse these with religious issues. Religious preference is something different, and personal to the individual, and, therefore, I talk little of this. Some prefer to leave religion alone, others take their religion seriously indeed and it is our experience that, whatever their choice, people explore that avenue for themselves. The techniques talked about in this book have no religious loadings, nor do they interfere or impose on patients' preferences in any way. However, the majority of people do find the techniques an aid in their search for their own Spiritual Reality.

Most people, and cancer patients in particular, are concerned with the basic questions: Who am I? What *is* life? Where did I come from? and Where am I going? These fundamental spiritual questions are often foremost in a cancer patient's mind and are certainly worth exploring in a public forum.

In these pages we shall consider also the increasingly recognised role that environmental and psychological factors play in the causation and treatment of cancer, for herein lies the key to success. We *can* identify the majority of the causes of cancer. I contend that there are also techniques available to deal with those causes. The techniques centre on appropriate diet, positive thinking, stress management and meditation – all in conjunction with suitable, specific therapies. By utilising all these means, the body's natural healing urge can be helped to reassert itself.

A body with properly functioning defences cannot have cancer.

Grace and I have experienced the pleasure of working with other patients who have been able to repeat the process that we went through and become free of an otherwise terminal illness. But the most exciting and pleasing aspect of our work is that the techniques we use have so consistently produced in patients a deeper love for life coupled with a profound acceptance of the outcome of that life.

So, while we have seen and continue to see many recoveries, we accept that not all patients are going to become free of their physical problems and that some will die. But it has been part of our joy to know that those who used the same techniques but did not recover were able to die with great dignity and poise that often surprised and always impressed themselves and their families. In this way, too, cancer was truly conquered. So although we always aim to help patients back to full health, our approach is of great value to those in a terminal condition who face dying.

While in general the earlier in the course of their illness a patient begins using our approach, the easier they will find it and the better their result, there is for those making a later start still the real prospect of overcoming cancer. There are always genuine grounds for hope, plus the bonus of overcoming fear and the problems associated with the disease. For many others there is the exciting prospect of using this approach to prevent cancer. We have found that you can, indeed, conquer cancer.

There were two main aspects to my recovery. These were the tremendous outside help I received and the inner resources I was able to mobilise.

Many individuals contributed to my recovery. My wife Grace played the most significant role by far. If everyone could have a person in their life so capable of showering total, loving care on them as Grace has for me, disease would be a thing of the past. She has shared in all my trials and efforts and, most importantly, right from the start she always *knew* I would get better. No doubts – she knew – and remained devoted to helping me do it. As many have found since, she has a wonderful ability to determine what is the right thing at the right time.

There were many others: Dr Ainslie Meares with his tremendous insight and his innovative meditation technique that is a major contribution to the health and well-being of the world at large, and cancer patients in particular; Pat Coleby who introduced me to Steve and Annette Henzler, who introduced me to the Gerson diet; Mike Sowerby who has enlarged and encouraged my interest in dietary considerations; my surgeon, John Doyle, who is a man of compassion; the psychic surgeons in the Philippines; Alan Mendizaba; Norma; Peter Hoddle; Jo Johansen and her Hobart friends; the Reverend Mario Schoenmaker; Dick Molesworth; Ralph Thomas; Bob Allen; Maurice Finkel; Ivan Burns; Mary Rogers; Pamela and Hari Bhagat; Sai Baba; the Findhorn community; my family and our many friends – the list goes on, and each contributed their part. What I hope to do is to amass their information in one place. My healing has been a gift from many others and overall from the Divine.

Of my inner resources, I feel the most significant was an ability to see the disease as a process. As soon as it appeared, I felt that it was a product of my past actions. Recognising that I had been involved in causing it, I felt confident that I could play a major role in getting over it. I accepted responsibility for my condition and therefore I felt in control of it. I was convinced that if I took the appropriate action, I would be cured. It then became a matter of making the appropriate changes in my life and finding the techniques to effect those changes.

For the benefit of others, I offer this book.

A final word

There is no magic bullet in this book. No wonder drug or herb that can be taken three times daily and which, leaving all else unchanged, will offer you a cure.

You *can* conquer cancer using a process – a healing process which takes effort, perseverance, and does require changes to be made. It is a process through which our natural state of health can be regained. For those prepared to walk this road I know that cancer can be prevented or overcome. My wish is that more and more people will do it.

Ian Gawler,
March 1984

Chapter one

THE FIRST STEP

For those willing to take up the challenge that cancer has put to them, there *is* a road back to health. The chapters of this book will discuss the options along the way. It is intended to help you make the right decisions for yourself and give you the motivation to persevere.

But where to begin? What is the first step? It is important at the outset that I say: 'There is nothing that *I* can do for you. It is a matter of what *you* can do for *yourself.* You can cure yourself – I am sure that is possible. However, all I can do is to show you the techniques and light the way.'

The starting point is having hope. You must be courageous enough to take the first step – then the rest will follow. We are seeing many people overcoming their problems and, in fact, becoming what the Americans call 'weller than well'. People who have been through this ultimate challenge of facing a life-threatening disease and emerging victorious feel a new zest for life, a new joyousness. They experience life as never before. You, too, can do it. It does require commitment and effort on your part; it can be hard work. Take heart, it can be done! But first sort out your priorities. If your illness has just been diagnosed, I suggest there are four questions you should consider:

Question 1   Do I really want to get well again?

You may say I am crazy to ask a question like that. The fact is, many cancer patients do accept their condition as terminal and cannot see themselves getting well again. They need either to change their attitude or to be prepared to concentrate on making the most of the time which they consider left to them. For the latter people, quality of life is of paramount importance and that should include preparing for a dignified, comfortable death. As explained in the introduction, the principles about which we will be talking have also proved to be of great help to the dying.

There is, however, a great deal of evidence providing the grounds for belief in a recovery from cancer, and that is our preferred objective. Cases such as my own and others of our Support Group, the books and reports of Ainslie Meares, the Simontons in the United States and workers in England, all reinforce the possibilities.

There is no doubt that those techniques described are effective. So, presuming the basic will to live is there, and remembering that a great deal can be done to build it up, we go on to:

Question 2   Do I want to take responsibility for my own condition?

This question is best characterised by imagining a visit to your doctor. Do you go to him and say, 'Here is my diseased body. You fix it. You tell me what is wrong. You decide what treatment I will have. I will accept whatever you say. The responsibility is yours'?

Or, do you go to him and say, 'Here is my diseased body. What can we do to get it better again?' With this latter approach, the relationship becomes a more equal one. Instead of handing responsibility for your well-being – and your life – to someone else, you are embarking on a shared quest for health. It implies that you *will* be informed – to the best of your ability to understand – as to just what *is* your situation. The full range of possibilities will be presented to you and, quite naturally, the professional's considered opinions and suggestions offered. But, the ultimate responsibility will remain with you.

I want to make it clear that I do not decry the medico's role. The doctor should be the central figure in dealing with such a major disease. I do feel strongly, however, that patients should be willing and able to accept responsibility for their own condition and treatment. I view abuses of this situation as either weakness on the patient's behalf or over-defensiveness on the part of the doctor.

Grace and I are often asked by patients what they should do in a given situation. If we can give a range of options we do so happily, but we always turn such questions back to the patient. All decisions must be the patient's, and we then urge total commitment to those choices. For this reason decision-making is discussed at some length later in these pages.

Question 3   Which should I use, toxic or non-toxic therapies?

Toxic therapies
Those that involve damage to the body
Surgery – does not necessarily affect the rest of the body
Radiation – damage can be localised
Chemotherapy – often affects many areas of the body

Non-toxic therapies
Those that do not cause damage
Meditation
Dietary considerations
Positive thinking
Immunological stimulants
Vitamin/mineral therapy
Wide range of so-called alternative therapies

This is the really hard question. It is a fact that most of the conventional therapies are toxic to the body. Radiation, and chemotherapy especially, frequently impair the body's own immune system, that is its *defence* mechanism. This reduces the body's ability to heal itself. Often this impairment is severe and side-effects can be marked. Radiation burns, vomiting and loss of hair are common, obvious problems that can follow. The impact on the rest of the body can be and often is less obvious, but never-the-less more drastic in nature. Minor infections that previously would have been of no consequence can assume major proportions. Most importantly, the body's own ability to fight the cancer is frequently lessened. This aspect of such treatments requires careful consideration. To my mind, it means that if you are having a toxic form of therapy, it is all the more important to concentrate on those self-help techniques which do aim to boost the immune system and help the body to help itself. These techniques are discussed in later chapters.

Here again, good communication with your doctor is essential. You must be able to discuss all your concerns freely and easily with your main doctor. If this is not the case, talk with that doctor about it. We all know some personalities clash and there are some people you just do not seem able to get along with. If you cannot find a way to correct the situation, then request a referral to someone more suited to your temperament. No one should be offended by this. It will make life easier and more constructive for everyone.

Similarly, it is sensible to weigh the possible benefits of any treatment against any possible side-effects of that treatment. The only logical way to do this is by comparing statistics. However, bear it in mind that statistics are notoriously inaccurate, especially when attempts are made to apply generalisations to specific, individual cases. Most doctors now avoid giving cancer patients a definite prognosis, or time of life expectancy, as there are so many variables. Frequently these 'sentences' prove to be so very wrong. However, one can get a good guide to the relevance of a specific form of treatment from such broad statistics. For example, in my case, when the cancer reappeared the range of life expectancy was three to six months. Conventional treatments offered little hope of altering that statistic and their side-effects would have been severe. It was easy for me to turn my back on them and to explore the other possibilities. If I had happened to have Hodgkin's Disease the situation would have been very different. Chemotherapy frequently cures this form of cancer, so in that case, on balance, any side-effects would have been worth considering.

The logical way to assess any proposed form of treatment would be to ask the following questions about it:

(a) What does the future hold for you if no treatment is given, and in such circumstances what range of life expectancy would you have?

(b) What range of life expectancy would you have if given the proposed form of treatment?

Note: These statistical ranges should be available in virtually all but experimental situations. If they are not provided upon request, I would be suspicious and seek another opinion. If you are considering an experimental treatment, you can only assess it on its possible merits. In other words, *you need to know* the anticipated benefits of the treatment.

(c) What are the side-effects of the treatment?

With these questions answered you have the basis for a decision. You can weigh the advantages against the disadvantages.

You may still have a very difficult decision to make. The non-toxic therapies with no side-effects have instant appeal, but they do not have the support of the medical mainstream as a first-line treatment. There is a growing number of doctors who are keen to utilise them where appropriate. They also recognise that these non-toxic therapies, such as diet, meditation and positive thinking, can be added as supportive measures for the more usual toxic therapies. Patients who do use them get less side-effects; furthermore, they do respond significantly better and, most importantly and dramatically, they have a far better quality of life. We see this consistently in the Melbourne Cancer Support Group where most people are having conventional therapies of one form or another.

Some other people, however, have either not been suitable for toxic therapies or have chosen the non-toxic therapies as their first choice. It takes courage to opt for something that frequently is described as experimental or, worse, as quackery. Again, however, the evidence is steadily accumulating that these therapies do stand in their own right and as time goes on they will be better evaluated and more widely utilised.

The choice remains difficult, but one that should be made consciously, preferably before any treatment commences. Once made, the final question follows:

Question 4   Which specific therapies shall I use?

Once the previous three questions have been answered, this one can be decided fairly easily. To have answered Question 3 well, implies close contact with the appropriate practitioners. Once you have clarified the issues and are to this level of commitment, you can feel confident to go along with their specific recommendations. So, for example, if you decide to have chemotherapy, it is reasonable to leave the choice of agents to be used to the doctor. You may desire, however, to know more or less of the details of your treatment and you should expect to have your questions answered in an open, cooperative manner.

Alternatively, if you were to choose meditation, you would need to commit yourself to learning the techniques and devoting the specified time to its practice.

Whatever the final choices you make, the next step is to do all that you possibly can to make sure the treatment works to full effect. We will discuss the means to achieve this throughout the book.

To the Medical Profession

In cancer there are many difficult questions to ask and answer. Often in the past the issues have been clouded by emotions and misunderstandings. I am well aware of the deep waters we are entering. Likewise, I trust it is obvious that I feel no conflict with the profession. I have been deliberating upon the contents of this book for some seven years and working actively with cancer patients for three years. I feel it is time to stand up and be counted. I accept the responsibility that this entails. I only ask that you endeavour to assess these principles with an open mind and let your judgement be influenced by the results they achieve.

No doubt you have all seen two patients with similar conditions. Given the same treatments, one responds, the other does not. Why?

Often you of the medical profession have concerned yourselves primarily with things that you could do for, or to, the patient, those external things that aim to destroy the symptoms of disease. I am sure that this contribution is vital, but it does not take into account the patient's input. Also, while some external, toxic therapies are useful, for the majority of cancers survival rates remain unimproved despite the enormous research efforts of the last twenty to thirty years. A broader perspective is required. Patients frequently feel that their quality of life is reduced by toxic treatments – and to what avail? Often they feel as if their quality of life is not even considered. Patients cannot be treated like a piece of machinery that is expected to respond to repairs in a standard way. Doctors need to be much more than body mechanics.

The patients' belief system, their hopes, fears, expectations and their level of well-being, all drastically affect the outcome of any treatment. They, the patients, can make the difference between success and failure.

Patients can be taught to achieve success. There is a better way. It involves mobilising the patient's own resources.

Over half the patients attending our Support Group are referred directly by doctors so I trust this book will allow for an even wider appraisal by those in the medical profession of the techniques we use.

To those interested in prevention

My wife, Grace, shared in all these techniques, doing all that I did. She was basically well to begin with. Now her level of health, her vitality, her capacity to give out, her joy for life, are increased manyfold.

If you are well, how well? Are you just symptom-free, or are you as fit as your true potential allows?

One in three people alive in the United States today will get cancer during their lifetime. One in five in Australia will die from it. This is not scare-mongering. This is fact. Are you prepared to learn the lesson of this disease and take up on a lifestyle aimed for optimal health?

These techniques that we talk of can save cancer patients' lives. We have seen them work for many other disease conditions as well. They can make a normal person a picture of health. In his work, *The Causes of Cancer*, Professor R. Doll gives the claim of medical authorities that 85 per cent of all cancers could be prevented by changes in lifestyle.[1] The challenge is there. It takes effort, it requires commitment and an ability to be open to change. Again, it can be done. Our natural state *is* health. Please take up that challenge. It would be wonderful to see people learning from the difficulties of others and not having the need for change forced upon them by physical disease.

Life was meant to be easy. And joyful. We just need to relearn those simple truths that make it so.

Chapter two

MEDITATION

The principles behind the silent healer

Meditation is the single most powerful tool to aid recovery from disease and lead to a life of maximum health. It provides all the basic ingredients. It has direct physical effects ranging from relief of physical tension to reactivation of the immune system. It aids the development of emotional and mental poise, generates a positive attitude and, most importantly, leads automatically and effortlessly, to a heightened level of well-being. Little wonder that it is enjoying such a rise in popularity as a self-help technique! When coupled with dietary considerations and active efforts to utilise the benefits of positive thinking, it forms the pillars upon which to build total health.

In the past, meditation has been used by most major religions as one part of a complex five-step process intended for developing a heightened level of consciousness. Today the word 'meditation' means different things to different people. Currently 'meditation' is used to describe many quite different processes, one of which is a technique for achieving deep relaxation which is now used as passive therapy for health purposes. Since this technique is not involved with direct spiritual endeavour, and also to avoid confusion in the text, the particular form of passive meditation that we use in this healing context will be expressed in italics, i.e. *meditation*, while that other kind of meditation that forms part of the five-step spiritual process will not be italicized.

We must remember that it is only in the last twenty years or so that medical innovators like Dr Ainslie Meares have identified the health promoting possibilities of the ageless forms of meditation and applied them to modern, everyday problems. Dr Meares' first major contribution in this area was popularised in his best-seller *Relief Without Drugs*.[2]

Dr Meares recognised that the benefits of *meditation* really flowed on from a point of stillness. A still mind, in a still body. He found that in this stillness the body has the opportunity to return to its natural state of balance. He also found that, if practised regularly, the refound state of balance persisted throughout the day, helping the patient to return automatically to that condition of balance we call health! Just as a cut finger heals itself automatically without us dwelling upon it, so passive *meditation* can reactivate natural healing mechanisms which operate automatically and have profound effects. It is to his great credit that Dr Meares was able to perceive this and then devise a simple means of leading people to that point of stillness and balance without, say, twenty years of rigorous concentrated study and practice of Zen discipline.

As a psychiatrist, his first experiments with such techniques began by helping people to cope with anxiety and stress-related problems. The more areas he tackled, the more successes he discovered. He soon found that *meditation* relieved such diverse symptoms as phobias, high blood pressure, allergies, nervous tension and pain intolerance.

This may sound extraordinary, but when we understand the nature of stress and the role it plays in so many disease situations, the reasons behind it become obvious. Having an understanding of how stress affects us, makes it easier to grasp how our present situation has arisen and provides us with a vital clue in planning our self-help program. So to understand just how stress affects us, let us look at the simple case of what happens when we get a sudden fright: Suppose that a bolt of lightning were to hit the ground near where you were standing. Your body would react quickly, almost instantaneously. With a gasped, 'Oh!' you would take a sharp breath and your muscles would contract with a jerk. Your body chemistry would change instantly as hormones were released. Adrenalin would flow and cortisone levels rise. Your heart would race, your blood pressure increase and your blood would be diverted to the muscles of action. You would have been readied for immediate action, thanks to the automatic changes produced by what is called the 'fight-or-flight' response. In our example, if you were quick you would have dived under cover. Then you would have realised that it was only lightning, that it had missed and everything was all right. 'Ahh!' would have come the response. The tension would be released and you would relax.

The events in this sequence are very important. The challenge gave rise to a bodily reaction which immediately prepared you for physical action. There followed a period of physical activity which was consummated and in turn followed by release. The sequence can be summarised:

Challenge

Bodily reaction with changes in body chemistry

Appropriate physical action

Release

It is a perfectly healthy sequence that was developed in earlier times when life was simple and very physical in nature. The fight-or-flight response was then a vital aid for self-preservation. So if the man in the cave next to yours came running over the hill with a club in hand, intent on stealing your wife, the threat was obvious. It produced rapid changes in body chemistry and you were immediately prepared for action. This would lead on to your doing the appropriate thing. If you felt you had a chance, you stood your ground and fought it out; if not, you ran. Either way, the challenge was resolved by a period of intense physical action which was followed through to a definite conclusion. You would then be free to relax, either licking your wounds or basking in success.

This sequence flowed with the rhythm of a simple life and it left no hang-over effects. Any fears that did remain were healthy ones based purely on instinct and self-preservation. Such fears did little to lessen the quality of life or lead to any physical symptoms. Animals in their natural state still demonstrate the appropriateness of this fight-or-flight response in a physically orientated world.

However, for we humans living in modern times things are no longer so simple. The challenges we face now are rarely of a purely physical nature and frequently are complex indeed. Most, if not all of our challenges nowadays are emotional or mental in their origins. However, an even greater problem is that frequently they are difficult to resolve.

So, whether it is a difficulty with a relationship or a financial worry that concerns us, it is easy to experience the same physical response. When the boss is overbearing and demanding or the neighbour disturbs our sleep early on Sunday morning with his lawn mower, we react in the same old way. We take that short little gasp and tense our muscles. Our body chemistry changes rapidly, preparing us for action. But can we punch the boss's nose or wrap the neighbour's mower around his ears? Not if we want that pay we need to meet our commitments, and not if we want to remain socially acceptable in our community! Often then, taking action is inappropriate and so our response is stifled. Now every time we face that same situation, or even think about it, the unresolved tension is reinforced.

Worse still, we frequently do take what seems to be the appropriate action and, even so, the situation remains unresolved. There is no obvious conclusion, no release, no return to basic body chemistry. We are locked into a situation where the changes in body chemistry persist.

Those changes in body chemistry associated with the fight-or-flight response are fine in the short term. They are an appropriate preparation for a short period of intense activity. They are not appropriate for long periods and they are not appropriate for maintenance.

If these changes to our body chemistry persist, we experience what is known as stress. Stress is a challenge that leads to a prolonged untoward effect on a person. *Stress occurs when there is an inability to take appropriate action in response to a challenge and so release it.* Therefore, stress is an unresolved challenge.

It is easy to appreciate that stress is a very personal thing. It is really determined by how we *respond* to a challenge, rather than by the nature of the challenge itself. What may be an easily resolved challenge for one person may produce profound stress for another.

The next key is that persistent stress affects the body chemistry in such a way that the body's immune system is depleted. It is particularly those changes in hormonal levels that reduce the body's ability to maintain and repair itself. And so, with time and other factors such as poor diet, stress leaves the way open for many diseases to precipitate. The American Academy of Physicians states that stress related symptoms lead to two-thirds of all visits to American family doctors. Stress is a major contributor, either directly or indirectly, to absenteeism, coronary heart disease, lung conditions, accident injuries, cirrhosis of the liver, suicide and a host of lesser ailments. I am convinced that stress is a major causative factor in cancer.

Virtually all cancer patients I have asked recognise that stress was a major factor in the development of their disease. Most recognise that firstly there was a chronic level of stress in their lives. But, more importantly, they are generally able to identify with a common psychological profile of cancer patients. In about 95 per cent of patients asked, this involved one particularly severe stress experience precipitating a drastic drop in their well-being. The stressful event occurred long before their cancer was diagnosed, but its untoward effects continued. This highly significant factor will be discussed in detail when dealing with the causes of cancer in Chapter 9.

For the moment, though, how do you know when stress is a problem? If it is not patently obvious, as it often is, muscular tension is a good guide. If you suffer from stress, one of the body changes it will produce is physical tension. Your body can be your guide. If you are free of muscle tension, feeling relaxed and well, then no problems! If your brow is knitted, your jaw clamped shut, your shoulders rigid or your hands clenched tightly, if you feel physical tension – beware! It is a warning signal. With appropriate action you can avoid problems. Understanding the stress cycle makes it easy to understand how to deal with stress. It is not necessary to avoid it, just deal with it appropriately. *All you need is a means to release it.* All successful people who cope well with potentially stressful situations have their personal means of finding release, of relaxing, of letting go.

But the easiest, the safest and the most reliable method – the best method for relieving muscular tension and stress – is passive *meditation*. Because *meditation* concentrates simply on a profound relaxation of the body and mind, it provides the opportunity for release – it allows us to let go!

The release found in the initial, formal periods of meditation soon flows on to become part of our life. As we return to a more relaxed state, we return to basic body chemistry. With that, our body is able to maintain and repair itself again and we have satisfied the first essential for a return to health – we have the body helping!

So if you are aware of mild levels of stress, but have no symptom of disease, short periods of *meditation* will cope with it quite readily. A life without challenge would be dull and lack zest, but we do not want challenges to become stresses – they should remain as opportunities. *Meditation* is a wonderful way to turn stress into opportunity.

If you do already have a disease problem, then longer periods of *meditation* will be indicated.

So now we can tabulate the role stress plays in disease:

The role of STRESS in Health and Disease

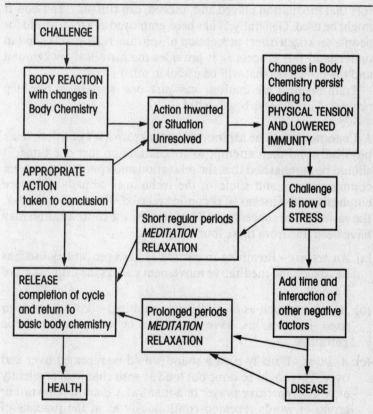

Once we understand this cycle, we can understand why *meditation* for health should be so simple and uncomplicated, why it should involve the relaxation and release that comes with stillness.

For many people, then, *meditation* has been enough. Practised regularly, it frees them from the bondage of stress, allows them to relax and so enjoy life to the full. *Do* use this basic self-help technique and make it a part of your life. The benefits will repay the initial effort.

However, before you look at the techniques of *meditation* in detail, you may find it helpful to understand the more traditional role that meditation played and, indeed, can still play, and how it might be used. Generally, it has been employed as a tool, an aid for people seeking a direct perception of spiritual reality. It is good to understand this process as it provides the historical background and the principles that will be useful in other areas.

Traditionally, meditation was just one step in a five-step process. This process began with:

1 Concentration: The aspirant would take up a set position, relax physically and then attempt to concentrate on just one thing. It should be emphasised that the relaxation and concentration were complementary and some of the techniques actually did place emphasis on the means of becoming relaxed. The more you relax, the easier it is to concentrate. The focus for the concentration may have been one from these four categories:

(a) *An activity* – Breathing in particular has been widely used, as has dance and meditative movement such as the Chinese art of Tai Chi.

(b) *An object* (such as a candle or a painting) – Ikons have been used for this, as have mandalas or complex, symbolic paintings.

(c) *A sound* – Usually such a sound would be repeated over and over. This could be done out loud as with chanting, or silently as with a repetitive prayer or a mantra. A mantra is a word or group of words repeated continuously as in the practice of Transcendental Meditation (TM).

(d) *A thought* – Generally a particular quality would be

concentrated upon; truth, honesty, justice, are typical examples used.

Whatever the nature of the focus for concentration, the aim was to think of that focus and nothing else. Once this was achieved, meditation was under way.

2 Meditation then was the ability to concentrate on one thing to the exclusion of all other thoughts. It was an active process of the mind which required some effort. In this traditional sense, meditation was really undistracted concentration. When practised long enough it led on to:

3 Contemplation: In contemplation, the act of concentration became automatic and effortless. It was as if the mind slipped into overdrive. When this occurred, instead of the logical, thinking part of the mind being at work, the intuitive, creative aspect came into play.

It is important to recognise that the mind *does* have these two distinctive ways of functioning – one rational, the other abstract. Most of us are only familiar with the day-to-day rational processes of the brain. All day our brain is thinking, analysing, evaluating. We have a steady flow of thoughts from the time we first arise to the time when we lapse into sleep at night. This rational, mental activity is normally associated with the left half of the brain.

Normally, we would associate times of non-thinking with sleep or unconsciousness. However, we may have experienced fleeting moments of non-thinking consciousness in that pleasant reverie that sometimes descends just before sleep. This peace is similar to those wonderful moments when a glorious sunset or a major work of art touches our inner core and leaves us in rapturous silence. We are then involved with that more abstract, less rational brain activity which is associated with the right side of the brain.

Many of us, then, could be laughingly referred to as half-wits because, being rational creatures, we only use half our brain's potential! Contemplation is a way to exercise the other half. By doing so, fresh insights can be gained and new levels of meaning obtained. The mind, however, is still active during this phase of the process. In contemplation it is just being used in a way with which we are not normally familiar.

Prolonged contemplation leads on to a state of:

4 Unification: This is a still more abstract state. In it, the contemplater, the object of contemplation and even the act of contemplation merge so that there is no awareness of separation, just an abiding sense of unity. This union is what the mystics of all ages have sought so earnestly and waxed poetic about when they found. It led on to a final state of:

5 Illumination: This was described as "the Knowing that passed all understanding'. In this state, totally new information would appear 'out of the blue' – the true revelation.

We can see how this five-step process works if we use the example of concentrating on a candle. Initially, concentration is required to sit still and to focus the attention on a candle. The mind may want to wander – What is for tea? What am I doing tomorrow? Should I scratch my nose? etc.

Eventually, with persistence and effort, we can concentrate on the candle without being interrupted by other thoughts. This is meditation. Soon, it is as if another thought process begins and abstract thoughts of the candle become apparent. The symbolism of the candle, its shape, its light, its fire, may be reflected upon and their nature assumes a new level of understanding. This is contemplation. For example, you may feel as if the light of the candle is a symbol of the Divine Spark within yourself and feel enriched by this awareness. As time goes on such thoughts gently fade and all awareness of activity and time are lost. Only in retrospect can you be aware that you were in a state in which you felt at one with the candle. This is Unification. This sense of oneness may extend beyond the candle and your immediate environment to give a direct appreciation of your oneness with everything around you. This type of mystical experience puts a smile on people's lips that does not readily fade!

Finally, completely new information may come to your awareness with force and clarity. From contemplation of the candle you may have sensed the meaning of the Divine Spark; now, in Illumination, you may have direct Knowing that such a Divine Spark *is* within yourself and every one of your fellows. This Knowing is irrefutable. It is not the knowing gained through reading or listening to others. It is the Knowing of direct experience. It may not even be justifiable in rational terms; no worry, you Know it as Truth.

It is vital to appreciate that this process we have been discussing is an active one and very different from the type of *meditation* we use for healing purposes. The *meditation* used for healing must be passive, not active.

I had been fortunate to have my cancer at a time when Dr Ainslie Meares contemplated the use of *meditation* for cancer patients. I had an emerging interest in the traditional forms of meditation and felt that these principles should be able to restore the inner harmony which I felt I had lost. I felt that if I could regain that inner harmony it would be reflected on the outer physical level. Dr Meares' idea was that the *meditation* would relieve anxiety and stress. This would lead to a reduction in the levels of cortisone in my body and so allow my immune system to operate normally. Then my body would remove the tumours itself. It would return to normal. It all sounded good to me.

As I have practised it more and come to see others benefit from it, too, there appear to be two broad areas of benefit: *Meditation increases quality of life and quantity of life. People who do it feel better and live longer.*

Considering quality of life first, we see benefits on all levels of human experience. There are physical, emotional, mental and spiritual gains.

Physical benefits

Abnormal physical tension is a symptom of stress which we know inhibits the body's natural function. *Meditation* relieves physical tension. Many people are struck by how good their body feels once this tension is removed. They realise just how much tension they had before learning to *meditate* in this way. While they had come to accept it as normal, now they realise just how unpleasant it really was. Athletes have found that *meditation* can increase their performance, and certainly most people find their general efficiency in day-to-day tasks goes up extraordinarily. Consistently, heart rates go down, and even severely elevated blood pressure can return to normal. Dr Colin who joined our groups, not with cancer but as an interested observer, found that *meditation* and diet brought his severely elevated blood pressure back to normal in two months.

Emotional benefits

Emotionally, our own level of ease is greatly improved through *meditation*. People find they feel better about themselves. They feel more able to accept their limitations and to use their strengths positively. In so doing, they are more able to relate to other people in an open, honest and meaningful way.

Any cancer patient knows that being just that – a cancer patient – has its problems. Before cancer was diagnosed, you may have been a doctor, carpenter, housewife, whatever. To your friends you are now a cancer patient first and foremost, and everything else is a poor second. This can cause much awkwardness and can become quite a cause for anxiety in itself. It is remarkable how *meditation* leads to an acceptance of the situation and an openness that is infectious, putting everyone at ease.

For many people, *meditation* reduces any feelings of guilt and negative emotion. As a consequence, they develop a greater capacity for loving. While this often results in an improved quality of sexual love, it also improves that more erudite, selfless love and compassion for all. People find they are able to give of themselves more freely and so be of more help to those around them.

Mental Benefits

Mental anxiety, if present, hinders all aspects of our being. Its causes are endless, often unidentifiable. Frequently, psychiatrists have spent countless hours of trauma, raking over the past in a fruitless quest for the elusive cause of present anxieties. From the womb, to birth, the formative years, adolescence and beyond, all manner of incidents can be identified as potential causes for anxiety and stress. Even if the cause is identified, treatment often remains difficult.

There is a vivid example. The Lancaster bombers of World War II had their rear ends protected by tail-gunners. These men climbed into the tail section of the plane via a ladder. They lay down in the cramped fuselage and then had a perspex bubble slammed tight around them. Their only communication with the rest of the crew was by headphone. They then set off on an incredibly rough ride with little to dwell on except their solitary machine gun and the fact that on average they could expect to survive about two missions. An extremely obvious cause for anxiety. It was not surprising then to find that, after the war, those who did survive frequently felt great tension when they were confined in small spaces. Many of these found great difficulty in relaxing enough to produce anything when in the narrow confines of a toilet! They knew the cause of their problem, as did all who tried to relieve their anxiety. What happened? They invariably left the toilet door open!

There are two principles operating here: First, just knowing the cause of a problem is not necessarily enough to relieve it; an appropriate technique is also important. Second, if those men could not have related their inability to go to the toilet to their war-time experiences they would have felt a great deal more anxiety and suffered greater distress.

So, in seeking health, we need to understand as much about our situation as possible, as well as having appropriate techniques to deal with it.

It is a constant effort to live with the pressure created by persistent anxiety. It is like trying to keep the lid on a pressure-cooker all the time. It tires us physically, emotionally and mentally. Once that anxiety is relieved, we feel benefits all through, and our physical symptoms soon respond.

Perhaps Dr Meares' greatest contribution has been to show that *meditation* treats anxiety regardless of cause and, more importantly, it works even if that cause is unidentified. It does so by short-circuiting the stress cycle. It is a reliable means of passing quickly from those changes in body chemistry that are an integral part of the effects to stress, to release, and this heralds a return to normal function and health. This explains further why we should start the technique with relaxing the physical body and why 'release', or relaxation of body and mind, promotes a return to normal health, for once we return to that state of release, the body chemistry returns to normal and the normal state means *health*. Most excitingly, this return to health will occur regardless of the cause of the stress if only we can release it. This is what *meditation* achieves. Without needing to analyse or dwell on the past, it can take us easily and effortlessly on to enjoy refound health. All *we* need to do is keep the technique simple and uncomplicated, that is *let go!*

Spiritual Benefits

Spiritually, many people find that *meditation* leads on to a peace of mind they had not imagined possible. A member of our group, Glenyss, recently told me that her body had never been worse but that she had never felt so good! Her face was shining, full of enthusiasm, and she said she was experiencing a quality of life she had never known before.

This peace of mind comes at a level so fundamental that it becomes in reality a true, direct experience. Many people who have firm religious beliefs to begin with are surprised by the depth of this experience. While some are apprehensive that *meditation* may conflict with their beliefs, the usual experience is that it leads to a heightened appreciation of their particular religious leanings and a greater level of personal joy.

This experience is often even more noticeable in people with no fixed religious views. I am sure that we all would like confirmation that there is more to life than just this mortal coil. In the past, most people seem to have relied on the word of others that this was so. By contrast, in modern times there has been a common disenchantment with formal religion and an urge to seek direct experience. Frequently, however, as the immediate material world is explored more fully, it is found to be exciting, but lacking. There has to be something more. *Meditation* often leads on to a direct experience of that something more. You only have to see the smiles on the faces of some of our cancer patients to know that this is a reality.

Quality of life is fundamentally important. It has to be there to make life worth living. *Meditation* helps us to act appropriately on all levels. That, in turn, gives us a peace and joy that is a pleasure to behold.

But what of **Quantity of life?** How long am I going to live? That question can lurk in the recesses of our minds to catch our breath whenever we are unaware. If we are a cancer patient, that question can be a constant nagging fear unless we reach acceptance, unless we regain our peace of mind. This does happen.

There is plenty of evidence from the work of Dr Meares and people using similar techniques in the United States and the United Kingdom, that these techniques do increase quantity of life as well as quality. My own case attests to this and so do the lives of many of the people in our Support Group.

There is no doubt these techniques work. I once remarked to Dr Meares that I felt so good after having had this disease, that everybody should have it just to get those same benefits! I think I was a little carried away at the time, but the message is there. I now feel my whole quality of life to be vastly better than before I lost my leg. I *meditate* because I want to. I feel best if it is a regular part of my day. As Judy, another patient at the group said, recently, 'Cancer changed my life for the better. It has taught me so much and I have gained so much through it. I cannot imagine myself having done it all without the prompting cancer gave me.'

Chapter three

MEDITATION

Practising the art

How do we do it? How do we *meditate* in this way?

It is such a simple thing, this *meditation*, and yet we are used to great complexity in our modern lives. How do we re-learn simplicity? How do we learn to be still? How do we 'let go'?

It helps to understand something of the process. In *meditation*, we want the thinking brain to become still. We have already talked of the rational, analytical, thinking functions of the left side of the brain and the creative, intuitive, feeling aspect of the right side of the brain. In seeking explanations and in seeking to explain what it feels like, we are trying to use rational, left-sided thinking to elucidate an inherently irrational, but still very valid, right-sided brain activity. It is good, in fact mandatory, to seek such explanations, to be critical, to analyse everything we do, but to realise the limitations we face.

We can explain a great deal of the nature of *meditation*, how it works and what it does. But, please, appreciate that its true essence has to be experienced to be fully comprehended.

Dr Meares asked a venerated Yogi in Nepal what it was like to meditate. The Yogi replied by asking him how he would describe the taste of a banana. You can use words to make comparisons and descriptions, but in the end the only way someone else can really know that taste is to peel a banana and try it! It is a matter of direct experience.

I hope these words give you the impetus and the confidence to try *meditation*. I trust that they will leave you free to enter into this experience with an open, willing mind, knowing that you are embarking on a very personal, exciting venture.

I have felt *meditation* transforming my life for the better and I have seen it happen often in others. It is probably the most pleasant thing I can do on my own, and the most beneficial. It has a place in everyone's life.

As we set out then, we are aiming to still our body and our mind. We are seeking to reach a point of relaxation and release at a very deep, fundamental level.

The technique we shall use, begins with stilling the body. We then allow the experience of this stillness to flow on to our mind.

Let me explain: Firstly we use a fairly formal, dynamic procedure to relax the body. This is formal, in that we do it in a set way to begin with and dynamic in that, as we progress, the technique evolves to become a more flowing, more automatic one. We need to be open to the on-going principles of change and improvement.

Attitudes are most important. In modern society we are used to striving for achievement. If we want something we normally expect to have to work or struggle for it. Not so in *meditation*. Once we actually start the procedure, we need to abandon any sense of striving, for if we sit down to '*meditate* or bust', we can be sure of an unhappy result! The only striving may be in making the time to do it, exerting the will to say, 'This is my time for *meditation* and nothing else takes precedence.' That can be effort enough, but once we commence, the accent is on effortlessness. It needs to be an easy, passive process.

To reinforce the attitude that this is a health-promoting procedure, I find it helpful to begin with an affirmation. Nothing rigid or forced, just a gentle statement of intention, Usually, this is:

Let your eyes close gently.
Turn your thoughts inwards.
Remember, that this is a time for healing.

Some people feel comfortable in following with a prayer and this, too, can be beneficial. 'Not as I would, O Lord, but as Thou will', seems particularly appropriate. Then it is the stillness we seek.

The surroundings are also important when you are beginning. It is appropriate to be in as conducive an environment as possible. Ideally, you should feel secure, free from the prospect of interruptions and distractions, and be in a quiet, comfortable space.

A group of people all doing the same thing is very supportive, but *meditation* can easily be embarked upon in private.

Choose a room where you feel comfortable, that is one away from any bustle. If necessary, ask other people to leave you undisturbed. Be prepared to ignore the front door bell or telephone should they ring. Initially it is good to use the same place regularly and to practise at the same time each day, if possible.

Now, what position should we use. The position you choose only needs to satisfy two criteria – it should be a position that is symmetrical and a position that has an element of discomfort in it for you.

First things first. The symmetry is important as it enhances the feeling of poise and balance. It also adds to the technique a sense of formality, a 'specialness'. So, if we lie down, we would be flat on our back, arms loosely by our sides, hands palm up and loosely open. Our legs would be straight, just comfortably apart, and the feet would flop outwards. If sitting, we would have the feet flat on the floor, our back reasonably straight and our head either upright or supported by the back of the chair. The arms may rest on the arms of an armchair with the hands flopped over their ends. If the chair is armless, the hands can rest flat on the thighs or loosely cupped in the lap.

We can advance to squatting on the floor, free of support. There are many yoga positions put forward for meditation, with the most favoured being the Lotus position. Let it be stressed, however, that in the technique we use, no set position is required or given blanket recommendation. It merely needs to be symmetrical, a little uncomfortable for you.

Discomfort – why should we be uncomfortable to begin something that is going to be pleasant and beneficial? Using this technique, the mild, initial discomfort soon fades from our awareness. It is essential to begin with it, however, as it makes us concentrate more. This works to make the relaxation more profound. The more uncomfortable we are when we begin, the deeper our level of relaxation has to be for us to regain a feeling of comfort and ease. Please just try this as experience will soon show that this mild discomfort is an essential ingredient in the process.

Now we are ready to use our body as the tool to guide us into the experience of *meditation*. We do this by imposing relaxation on our body, feeling what that relaxation is like and letting it flow on to our mind. In the beginning we use a simple, formal procedure to capture that feeling. Once we have done that and can reproduce the feeling, we no longer need the formal technique. Remember that the emphasis of the technique is on feeling – an abstract, right-sided brain function.

We begin by closing our eyes and concentrating on feeling what our body is like when it is at rest. Then we impose tension upon it and feel the difference – the different feel our body now has. Then we relax the body and feel a third quality – that of deep relaxation. Finally we discover another state, what we call a 'letting go', when the body feels different again. Let me explain further.

We really need to experience this to understand it. Be assured, this is a very simple technique. By concentrating on one area of the body at a time we can feel what it is like; then make it tense, feel that difference, feel the tension, and then relax it. By repeating this technique through all the areas of the body we can quickly learn to relax the body very deeply indeed.

First we need to go through the different areas and learn how to feel them, impose tension on them and then relax them. We begin with the feet. Having taken up our chosen position, we let our eyes close gently and put all our attention on our feet.

When we do this well, we shift our centre of awareness. Normally, our centre of awareness is in our head, round about the space between our eyes. We feel as if that is the central point of everything for us. Now, by closing our eyes and concentrating on our feet, we feel as if they have become our centre. We then find that the feet just have a particular 'feel'. If you find that hard to realise at first, the second step makes it more obvious. You now contract all the muscles in the feet to impose tension on that area. In effect, you are making the feet rigid so that they are inflexible, immovable. The 'feel' is quite different. Feel that difference.

Next you let the muscles relax. You feel them becoming looser, softer. The more they relax, the heavier they feel. They feel as if they would melt down into the floor – like an ice-cream in the sun, gently melting. In deep relaxation, a feeling of warmth often accompanies this feeling of heaviness.

So there is the simple process. Feel the area, contract the muscles, and let them go.

As a first step, it is good to go through each area just to get used to contracting the muscles. Remember that this is an introductory technique, and that if you follow it you will soon experience *meditation* proper; then the technique loses its importance. You will then be able to go more directly into the *meditation*.

For now, begin by familiarising yourself with how to contract the different muscle groups. Sit symmetrically, let your eyes close gently, and contract the muscles of the feet. If you find the muscles hard to work, pull the toes back towards the heels while at the same time resisting any movement. This locks all the muscles tightly and gives a good impression of what tension is like in that area. Then relax the muscles.

The calves: Imagine someone was going to pull your ankle in any direction and you wanted to resist. This locks all the calf muscles as desired. You may notice some of the muscles of the thigh had to act also. Keep this to a minimum and concentrate totally on what is happening in the calves.

The thighs: These are the largest muscle group in the body and easy to feel the tension in. If necessary, try to lift the feet off the ground and hold the thighs down with the hands – the tension is then obvious.

The buttocks are contracted by squeezing the big muscles of the backside and so lifting a little off the chair. We want to be aware of the whole pelvic area, however, and feel the relaxation right through it.

The tummy: Here the need to feel the relaxation all through the area is more evident. We can contract the muscles of the tummy easily and we should include the muscles of the lower back as well. If we imagine that we are lying on our back and someone is about to drop a medicine ball on our tummy – the right muscles will be working! Then, when we relax, we feel the muscles relax and also feel all that is inside the tummy is relaxing as well. There is no need to try to imagine a relaxed liver, a relaxed spleen, etc. – just feel that same deep relaxation all through the area, in a general, non-specific way.

The chest: The same principle applies. We contract all the chest muscles and make it like a rigid barrel. Then we relax the muscles and feel the relaxation all through the chest.

The arms we do as one unit. Make them completely rigid as if resisting movement in any direction. Stiffening them produces the feeling of tension very readily; then feel the relaxation.

The shoulders (includes the throat region): Here we contract the muscles by lifting the shoulders and pulling the head down. Feel the relaxation then in the shoulders, neck and throat.

The jaw: Grit the teeth and feel the tension in the big muscles of mastication. Relaxing, feel it in the mouth, lips and cheeks, as well as the big muscles at the side of the jaw.

The eyes: Closing the eyes in a squint makes the tension obvious. Relax and feel it in the eyes and across the nose.

The forehead: Some people find it easier to frown than others! Contract the muscles, feel the tension, and let it go. Feel the forehead smoothing out.

The forehead and the hands are particularly important as over 60 per cent of the body's nerve endings are in these two areas. The more nerve endings we relax, the more we relax our brain; the more we feel the relaxation, the more we are truly relaxed.

Having become familiar with contracting the various muscle groups and relaxing them, we are ready for *meditation* proper. We need to go with this a little, to trust in its simplicity and allow ourselves to move into it. The body is the guide. As we feel it relaxing we feel our thinking processes winding down, and as the body enters the state of 'letting go' we allow the mind to flow into it, too.

As the body first relaxes, it begins to feel very heavy. It is so loose and relaxed, it feels as if it could just melt into the floor. Then, as it goes deeper into the process, it begins to enter a phase that we describe as 'letting go'. A new lightness comes over it. Often there is a tingling, a sensation of warmth, always a sense of comfort, pleasure and ease. If we let our mind go along with this feeling we soon lose all awareness of our body and surrounds. Noises seem far away and inconsequential, and we are left with an expansive, floating feeling.

I liken this feeling of 'letting go' to a sensation which is similar at first to floating peacefully in warm water. Then it is as if we were dissolving out into that water. Instead of the normal feel of our body being sharp and well-defined, in our mind, the edges start becoming fuzzy. We are used to feeling our hands, say, to be definite in outline. In *meditation* those barriers are not apparent. We

feel as if we are taking up more space than just the normal confines
of our body.

Back to the 'practicals'. To accentuate this technique based on
physical relaxation, we use simple abstract phrases to lead us
through the procedure. In the group situation, I lead this through
saying the words out aloud. At home you can begin by repeating
them noiselessly to yourself, or getting a tape with the words
recorded. The words should be repeated slowly and rhythmically.
Some people find it helpful to repeat one phrase every second
breath. That is, you breathe in; and say a phrase as you breathe
out; then breathe in again, breathe out, breathe in, and say another
phrase as you breathe out the second time.

You will find that as the relaxation progresses your breathing is
likely to slow down automatically. There is no need to emphasize
the breathing at all. It will adopt its own slow steady rhythm in a
natural way.

When contracting the muscles, hold the tension just long
enough to feel it strongly, then let it go.

So, if we get ourselves sitting symmetrically again, try these
words that I use:

Let our eyes close gently...
Turn our thoughts inwards...
And remember that this is a time for healing...
Turn our attention to the feet... really concentrate on the feet
... perhaps move them a little... really feel what they are like at
the moment... now contract the muscles of the feet... feel the
tension... feel the difference... and let them go... feel the
muscles relaxing... feel it deeply... completely... more than
relaxed... letting go... the calves... feel them... contract the
muscles... and let them go... feel it deeply... it is a good feeling... a natural feeling... feel it deeply... feel the letting go...
the thighs... contract the muscles... and let them go... feel it
all through... the legs feel heavy... as if they would merge into
the floor... more and more... letting go... the buttocks...
contract the muscles... and let them go... deeply... completely... more and more... deeper and deeper... letting go...
the tummy... contract the muscles... and let them go... feel
the tummy drop a little... it is a good feeling... feel it deeply

feel the letting go ... the chest ... contract the muscles ... and let them go ... feel it all through ... more and more ... deeper and deeper ... letting go ... the arms ... contract the muscles ... and let them go ... feel it in the hands particularly ... they feel heavy ... more than relaxed ... letting go ... the shoulders ... contract the muscles and let them go ... deeply ... completely ... more and more ... deeper and deeper ... letting go ... the jaw ... contract the muscles ... and let them go ... feel the jaw drop a little ... feel it deeply ... it is a good feeling ... a natural feeling ... feel the letting go ... the eyes ... contract the muscles ... and let them go ... deeply ... completely ... more and more ... letting go ... the forehead ... contract the muscles ... and let them go ... feel it in the forehead particularly ... feel the forehead smoothing out ... feel it all through ... more and more ... deeper and deeper ... letting go ...

After a period of silence, we usually finish by saying, 'That's good ... Let your eyes gently open now.'

And so what happens? Most people, on first doing it, are struck by the deep sense of physical relaxation it produces. They find this a new and exciting sensation which they want to repeat more often. Just recently, David, a cancer patient who is fifty-eight, said he had worked hard all his life and enjoyed doing so, but on trying this exercise for the first time, realised he had never before known the joy and pleasure of being so simply, deeply relaxed.

As people do it more, the stillness of the mind comes more rapidly and frequently. Do be assured that everyone can do this. Some people find their mind becomes still almost immediately; others need to persevere longer. Perhaps one of the most dramatic experiences was described by Jeff on his first occasion: 'I became so relaxed that I felt as if all my tension was drained out through my feet, leaving only an empty shell. Then it was as if someone came along with a huge pitcher of vibrant, fluid light. They poured this in through my head, making me feel sparkling and full of vitality. I have never felt anything like it before. I feel wonderful!'

Another lady, Madge, had trouble with persistent thoughts occurring, but stuck at it as she believed in the technique. After twelve weeks she came to me with a smile on her face and said, 'At last it is happening. I can feel it. I am finally experiencing times when my mind is still. It has been worth waiting for.' These cases show that there is a range of experience, and virtually everyone is different.

Thoughts are the most common difficulty. Nearly everyone can learn to relax their body in very short time – in one or a few sessions. I do feel that relaxing the body so completely plays a large part in the whole process, as it gets us well on the way to Release. Just achieving that physical stillness provides very significant benefit. While it is good to aim for a point where the mind is released also, it is important not to strive – not to try too hard for if thoughts do intrude, frustration can be a problem. It is a temptation to try to do battle with the thoughts and actively push them from our mind. This only strengthens them. We use the rational half of our mind in such attempts, and we want the rational mind to be still. We must be prepared to be passive, and patient.

If thoughts are continuing, we can briefly return to the body and do more relaxation, going over the body again using the key phrases. If we concentrate on the relaxation we feel in the body, we will feel it in our mind, and times of stillness will start to flow.

At the same time, our attitude to unwanted thoughts should be one of an uninvolved observer. We can understand this if we consider watching a film on television. If it is an action movie that has our full attention, we sit on the edge of our seat and identify so strongly with the film that it is as if we are a part of it. It becomes almost a real experience for us while it is on. If, however, it is late at night, we are tired and the film is old and dull, we sit back in our chair quite uninvolved with the action. We see the pictures moving around and we hear the sounds; but we are like a dispassionate observer.

If we can adopt that same attitude with unwanted thoughts, we give them no strength. If we allow them to just roll on, to come and to go, they do just that – and soon stop.

We must avoid frustration with any difficulties. Be assured they all do stop with time. This applies to all the common defence reactions that the body uses from time to time in an attempt to reassert itself. We must realise the body's main function is one of self-preservation, and in passive *meditation* we are introducing it to a very new and unfamiliar technique which carries with it a somewhat defenceless, open feeling. For most people this is an accept-able, in fact extremely pleasant, experience.

For some, and particularly (but not always) those in whom ten-sion is more obvious, the body and mind subconsciously object. So they might start the relaxation and feel a change beginning, only to be thwarted by an unwanted reaction. Some people feel a sud-den jerk throughout their body; others are struck with a sudden sense of panic. All these are defence reactions. They show that something really *is* happening – that you are in fact on the way to relaxing. All you need to do is to persevere. As you do it more frequently, your body and mind will adjust and allow you to pass this threshold and get on with the *meditation*.

On a more pleasant note, Harold, a sixty-three-year-old patient, regularly had sensations of seeing beautiful colours and images and hearing beautiful sounds. Some, like forty-eight-year-old Judy, become so relaxed that they even find themselves wonder-ing if their breathing has stopped. Others pass through a stage of rapid eye movements which feel like minor twitches. All of this is very interesting but tends to distract us from our purpose. If we get side-tracked by such phenomena, we miss the stillness wherein the best of the healing lies. It is simplicity and stillness we are seek-ing.

Remember that it is probable that you will have good sessions and bad ones to begin with. The more you do, the more repeatable it becomes.

Finally, then, what level of commitment is required – *quality of life* or *quantity of life?* Your aims and priorities must be very clear. Any time allocation has to be balanced by your needs, your beliefs and your other commitments.

Quality of life is vastly improved by doing ten to twenty minutes, two or three times daily. To make an impact on quantity of life, three sessions per day of around one hour each should be aimed for.

I feel it very important to set yourself a goal in this regard. Work out your priorities and set a goal for the next week. Ideally, at least three sessions per day works best. Decide how long you will aim to spend at each session. It is far better to set a conservative goal to begin with, and succeed in meeting it, than to fall short of an over-ambitious target.

So, having set your goal, practise for a week. Then assess your results, reassess your goals and priorities, and reset your target.

When I first began, my situation was critical and I did about five hours a day for three months. I then did three, hourly sessions for the next year, then around an hour each day ever since. This is obviously a big time commitment. I did it because it felt good and it gave me results. I continue to do around an hour each day for the same reasons.

If quality of life is your aim, and time appears short, ten to twenty minutes twice a day will help you a lot. However, remember the man who had been estimated to have three weeks to live. He went to Dr Meares full of enthusiasm for his ideas and keen to begin. However, on being told he would need to spend three hours a day at it he replied, 'Oh, I haven't time for that', and left!

I am sure *meditation* improves quality of life and quantity of life.

Only you can do it.

Chapter four

RELAXATION

The key to appropriate action

The body's natural ability to heal itself is really quite phenomenal. While we often take it for granted, this ability is nothing short of miraculous.

For example take the healing of a broken leg. First there is a trauma, a solid bone is broken in two and the shattered ends displaced. There will be torn muscles, probably internal bleeding – a lot of damage. Surgery is often required to stabilise the situation and perhaps a steel pin is inserted to fix the broken bones together and keep them stable. Yet, once the right conditions are created, that bone will automatically reunite itself, the muscles will regenerate and normal function return. In six months' time an X-ray will show the bone to be just the same as it ever was. What an amazing process!

Let us see this process in perspective. First, the right conditions were created, and then *the body healed itself.* The medical intervention was necessary to provide those right conditions. However, the doctors did not actually heal anything. All they did, by realigning the bones, was to create the first requirement for the healing of a fracture to proceed. The patient then had to look after the leg and make sure the healing process could continue. The patient did not have to think of the intricate process of the bones reuniting. The body's natural healing power simply returned the leg to normal. *The body healed itself* – automatically.

The body's normal state *is* health. It has a tremendously varied and complex set of mechanisms to maintain it in health. Whenever the body is out of balance, these mechanisms swing into action to re-create health. If those mechanisms are thwarted or unsuccessful, then we have disease.

So what is the problem in cancer? Why does the body appear unable to cope? It is just the same as with the broken leg! If we do provide the right conditions the body will heal itself.

In the acute situation of a broken bone, the medical intervention is a very obvious first step. Surgery provides the right conditions by realigning and stabilising the bones. The patient maintains those conditions by keeping the leg still and having a diet and environment which permits the normal healing functions to proceed. Cancer is a chronic situation, however. It takes a long time to develop and has a multiplicity of causes as we shall see in later discussion. Correcting these causes is more involved, and providing the correct environment to allow the healing to proceed is also more involved. It requires consideration of far more than the body mechanics involved in surgically repairing a broken leg. It involves consideration of the whole person.

What we are concerned with is looking at the patient's role in re-creating their own health. So what constitutes the correct environment for healing in general and cancer in particular? We are seeking a state of balance, a state of normalcy as the body's normal state is health, and health does not include cancer.

Again, a healthy body cannot have cancer. There was a man in America who had kidney failure and was given a kidney transplant. Unbeknown to anyone, the kidney he was given in the transplant was already cancerous. Naturally, he was on immuno-suppressant drugs to prevent his body rejecting this new kidney. This meant that his body's normal defences could not operate properly. In a very short time not only was the new kidney engulfed by the cancer but it had spread throughout his lungs. With his life threatened, the immuno-suppressant drugs were ceased, the new kidney was removed, and he was returned to a dialysis machine. What happened? His normal bodily defences rapidly re-asserted themselves and all the cancer in his chest disappeared – automatically, with no outside intervention. His body's normal ability to heal itself did just that. His body with its immune system working again, had the ability to recognise that the cancer should not have been there, and so removed it.

We want to allow our body to do that same thing. We want to reactivate our own immune system and provide the right conditions in which healing can take place. We can do it.

There is a very close link between the function of our body and the function of our psyche. That is, if we are relaxed and easy in mind and emotions, our body will be relaxed. If, on the other hand, we have anxiety or are affected by stress, our body will suffer from subtle but far-reaching changes in body chemistry and it will also show up physical tension. I believe that this reflex is a key factor which we can use in the process of getting well.

Equate stress, anxiety and tension with immuno-suppression
Equate relaxation with health

If our body and psyche are relaxed, we will be in a state of balance, and that balance means health. If we are deeply relaxed, our body's natural healing tendency will re-create health for us – true, deep, meaningful health, including a healthy body.

The first step, the starting point that we can readily appreciate and learn, is to get the body deeply relaxed. Relieving emotional and mental stress is hard to begin with as causes of anxiety are difficult to isolate and often difficult to treat using conventional means. If we relax the body, however, that reflex produces relaxation of emotions and mind.

Mental anxiety and stress, and physical tension, are intricately connected and inter-dependent. They are all disease-producing factors. However, truly break that connection at any one point, and relaxation spreads all through. Healing begins.

Pause to consider a cat. A lithe, graceful cat. Watch it on the move. It moves with an ease and smoothness that is a joy to watch. In slow motion it is a sight to behold. Yet if it has to react in a hurry, it can – in an instant. It will pounce in a flash, or turn and run with amazing speed. So, too, it will often stop, consider a situation at length, and then go on with its business. Concentration and relaxation are mutually supportive. All so easy, so relaxed. This, to me, shows what relaxation is all about. It is being physically relaxed and so being free to make an appropriate response.

If we are relaxed we react appropriately. We do not rush into things and over-react; neither are we sluggish and unable to take appropriate action. What we do is simply – appropriate.

There is no need to avoid the problems of everyday life. Life should have challenges and a zest of endeavour. Such challenges only become causes for stress when we do not handle them appropriately.

If we do not react to challenges well, tension and anxiety cloud our normal processes. They interfere with judgment and reactions, so that responses become inappropriate. The more relaxed our being, the more likely we are to do the appropriate thing. It is appropriate to have a healthy body, and a healthy body is a relaxed body.

Where, then, do we find this relaxation? The standard means of relaxation are sleep, exercise, hobbies and holidays. All have their place. Sleep is an excellent way of dealing with acute stress. Even sleep imposed by drugs will often provide the time and space necessary for adjusting to and dealing with a major, temporary stress. We certainly need a regular amount of natural sleep to avoid fatigue and added stress. We can improve the quality of our sleep by doing physical relaxation exercises when we go to bed.

When you get into bed at night, spend five minutes, perhaps ten, doing your relaxation. This is important. If you have muscular tension when you get into bed, your body is like a spring and you will spend half the night unwinding. Researchers have watched people sleeping and have seen the muscles of tense people struggling to unwind. In a series of jerks and twists, the body tries to get itself relaxed. For some people this might take all night and so they wake up without having much profitable relaxed sleep. So spend a few minutes before you go to sleep and practise the body relaxation. As you get that good relaxed feeling all through, you will find that you can put yourself to sleep. You could well find that you need less sleep than you used to, as well as waking feeling the better for it.

In chronic stress situations, however, sleep changes very little. We wake up with the same problems and responses that accompanied us to sleep. We need to look further.

Exercise is well worth considering. In the right amounts, it helps to relax physical tension by tiring the muscles and so creating a natural form of relaxation. Also, it certainly invigorates and makes the body feel better. We should have exercise as part of our health program, but still it does not change our basic condition.

Similarly with hobbies and holidays. They can be very pleasant diversions, they provide an opportunity to relax, release and let go a little. They can certainly aid our general level of well-being. They are well worth considering, but frequently they, too, produce little change in our overall situation. What then is left?

Obviously, the practice of *meditation*. Another reason why our *meditation* technique works so well is that it starts with a deep physical relaxation. Then, relaxing the mind enhances the effect.

Once we have learned to do that complete relaxation in our formal times of *meditation*, we start to experience the benefits of Release and return to normal body chemistry. The next step, then, is to be able to let the benefits of the *meditation* flow on into our everyday life. This is most important. The relaxation we feel during the *meditation* must become a way of life for us. We must aim to be as relaxed as possible because, except when we are faced with an immediate threat, relaxation is our hallmark of Release and normal body chemistry.

This is not to say we should be sluggish or lethargic. We can still react quickly and be sharp and alert, but, like the cat, be relaxed at the same time. There are a number of ways to achieve this.

As you begin *meditating*, you will notice that the calm you feel during it remains with you for a short while after. *Meditating* regularly in this way throughout the day enhances this effect, so that one session's benefits flow on to the next. This is why it is good to spread a number of sessions throughout the day. While initially you will seem to have good and bad sessions, soon you will notice a cumulative effect which means you get more benefit from each experience of *meditation*.

This effect can be increased still further by improving the quality of the *meditation* and by becoming more aware of relaxation throughout the day.

The technique that we use to achieve the stillness of the *meditation* must be seen as just that – a technique only, a means to an end. It is the quiet of the *meditation* we are seeking and the technique certainly will get us there. As time goes on, however, we should be speeding up the technique, even doing away with it.

Initially, then, we use the physical act of contracting muscles and letting them go. This produces a very deep relaxation and allows us to appreciate what it feels like to be deeply relaxed. The need to get the body well relaxed is the important starting point, but we will find that soon we can get that same relaxation, that same feeling of physical ease, without having to physically contract the muscles.

The next step, then, is to just think of the muscles in each area and feel them relaxing without having contracted them first. The endpoint still should be that same deeply relaxed body we felt with the first technique. Now, however, we are doing less to distract us. We have less to think of if we do not physically contract the muscles, and the ease of it all is more apparent. We are heading towards that ultimate point where we even do not need to spend time on individual areas. We can just sit down and feel a wave of relaxation move throughout the body, producing that total, deep calm.

However, there is no hurry in speeding up the procedure. We should feel confident at each phase before advancing. The accent is on ease. No effort, no striving, just a natural progressing to a faster, easier way. Again, the point to emphasise is that the body should be deeply relaxed, and so should the mind.

Once we find the procedure is working well, there is another step forward. Now we can begin to use a more uncomfortable starting position.

What, more discomfort? Yes, just a little at a time, because if that element of discomfort is there it makes the physical relaxation a little harder to achieve. It makes us focus more on what we are doing and, undoubtedly, it heightens the effect of the *meditation*. You really must try this; the results will be obvious.

If you began in an armchair, once the technique is working well try it in an armless chair. The change is very little but I am sure you will notice a different effect. Once you are comfortable with that and it has become easy and effortless, go on to trying it on a stool. Harder still, but still fairly easy and, again, a greater benefit. Then you could go on to squatting on the floor, or going outdoors. In the open air the sounds and smells increase the naturalness of it and, again, add to the effects.

In my own situation, I generally *meditate* squatting on the floor or on a chair in the morning and lunchtime. My back can often be tired after a day on one leg, so frequently I lie on a hard surface in the evening as this allows it to relax better. I notice that lying down produces more benefit in terms of relaxing my body, but there is no doubt squatting produces a better overall effect.

Another technique I use for getting the body deeply relaxed involves incorporating visualisation with the *meditation*. I make sure I do this as a separate exercise to the normal passive *meditation*. It is an optional extra, if you like.

In the book, we discuss other ways of meditating, visualising and contemplating. If you choose to use these extra techniques, do be sure that you use them separately from the passive *meditation*, for they are quite different.

For its effect, the standard passive *meditation* relies upon its simplicity and stillness. If we were to start using our mind actively in *meditation*, it then, of course, would be a completely different thing. However the active mind is another of our great resources and can be put to good use. So visualisation, which does involve the mind in an active way, has a place and can be added to the overall programme. Please do realise, however, that it is the passive, still *meditation* that has the primary role to play.

Practise passive *meditation* first and practise it well. When it *is* going well, and *if* you feel you could or want to do more, *then* consider these extras.

I cannot over-emphasise this. For health purposes, stillness is more appropriate than mental gymnastics. This understood, visualisation with the bodily relaxation can produce a greater depth of relaxation and an increased vitality. It also has the great advantage of leading on to a heightened body awareness. Using this technique you will be in better touch with your body and more responsive to its messages. Similarly, you will be able to control it better.

I call this the 'radiant light' visualisation. To begin, allow yourself at least thirty minutes. Visualisation can be done in any position, but I find this one works best if you lie down on a hard surface. The floor is ideal. Choose a carpeted area, or place a blanket underneath yourself to begin with. Lie flat on your back, hands loosely by your sides. Legs should be out straight, just comfortably apart, and the feet allowed to flop loosely outwards. Now put all your attention on to just one big toe. Form an image of it in your mind and travel through it, looking closely at each part, relaxing it as you go and feeling that relaxation. Travel around the skin, under the nail, through the joints, tendons, ligaments and muscles. You will find you can see it all quite clearly and produce a profound feeling of relaxation in it. As you do so you will notice it becomes a little warmer. It may tingle a little. Gradually you then build up the image of a glowing white light suffusing it all. It is as if that toe was a light globe with a dimmer switch. You turn on that switch and gradually increase the light until the toe is full of vibrant white light. You will find it feels marvellous. When you do it well, you will be thinking of nothing else, just experiencing the vibrance of it all.

In effect you are using the five-step active meditation process with your own body as the focus of attention. You concentrate on your big toe, actively meditate upon it being relaxed, contemplate it, and while it is filled with vibrant white light, feel unified with it. It may sound strange to feel unified with your own toe, and with your whole body as you extend the process, but it is not. In this state of true unity and true balance lie harmony, healing and health. If you hold this feeling it has very positive effects.

So, begin with one toe. Then move to the next, and so on, until the whole foot is 'lit up'. You may find that at the first session doing one foot takes all your time. That's fine. Next session you will find that you can recapture the feeling in that foot more easily and so can start with the next foot. At each session work on more areas until you can capture the feeling throughout the body. It is the feeling of relaxation, lightness and vitality that is the main thing. When you can do it well, you will have a means to relax yourself deeply and revitalise yourself amazingly. Practising this technique regularly, once a day for a few weeks, will produce a new dimension in body awareness and relaxation.

The clarity of visualisation of the different body parts is not so important. Obviously, someone with detailed anatomical knowledge will be able to build up a more detailed image than others. The important thing is to feel that close contact and awareness of each part of your body. So, in a large complex area such as the abdomen, you feel as if your mind is moving through the whole area. You feel the deep sense of relaxation and then the glow.

When it comes to areas affected by cancer or other disease, just do the same thing. No effort or striving, just feel your mind moving through the area, relaxing it and letting the light build up to the same level as in the rest of your body. This produces a feeling of uniformity throughout the body – a vital, healthy uniformity, and it promotes the healing response.

Sometimes, relaxing areas affected by disease causes some initial discomfort. This is because we often impose tension in the region around them as a defence mechanism. These exercises relax that tension and often produce sensations of temporary discomfort, occasionally tingling, even brief muscle spasms or jerks. Be assured this soon gives way to a feeling of warmth and ease and that this technique is also very helpful for pain control. [See Chapter Six]. Again, the aim of the exercise is to lead us to a point of profound relaxation, with an accompanying sense of wholeness and vitality. So it really serves to add another means of reaching the stillness of passive *meditation*. It is that end point which is the really important thing.

This visualisation exercise also puts us in better contact with our body so that we can appreciate better our level of relaxation through the day. Relaxation is one of our aims, and how much of it we feel through the day is a guide to our progress. The more relaxed we are, the better our progress.

As you become more aware of your body, you will almost certainly find that some areas feel more tense than others. Common areas of tension are the muscles of the forehead, jaw, shoulders, hands and lower back. You will find that when you are placed in a stressful situation, one or more of these areas may tense up first. Just watch what happens next time you are 'pushed'. These areas are called trigger areas and they are very useful! Remember the reflex?

Anxiety + Stress = Muscular tension

Muscular relaxation = no anxiety or effect from stress

Having identified localised areas where tension shows up, we can concentrate on relaxing those areas, and if we succeed in doing so we are well on the way to being relaxed. This is a very good defence mechanism to use if you feel stress is still affecting you. If you feel a situation is causing stress to build up, concentrate on relaxing your trigger areas. You will find that if you keep your body relaxed, the whole situation will be defused. Once you have experienced the 'feel' of relaxation in your formal exercises, you will be able to recapture it at will during the day. Soon it becomes your natural state. Free from tension, you will be able to react appropriately and will not be affected by stress.

Ideally, we want to be relaxed all day and impervious to potentially stressful situations. Practising these techniques goes a long way towards this end and we can do still more to achieve it. At every opportunity through the day, at every idle moment, take the time to check your level of relaxation. Do an internal inventory. Start with the trigger areas and make sure that they are relaxed. To begin with, you may find that every time you think of them they need to be relaxed more. That's fine. Relax them with a smile, knowing that the worse the tension to begin with, the more benefit you will get in the long run by relaxing!

Seek to experience the feeling of relaxation at every opportunity. After a while you will stay relaxed and you will feel a wonderful difference.

So use your time wisely. When in the car, don't just waste those precious seconds at the red lights. Relax as much as you can and feel how good it is. Even while driving along, be aware that your trigger areas are relaxed and then that the rest of your body feels good also.

The key to this is the principle that you should only use the muscles you need for any given task of the day. Muscles should either be working at a specific function or at rest. There should be no residual tension. Think of this with the cat. As we watch him in slow motion his foreleg flows gracefully forward. All the muscles at the front of his leg are contracting to draw the leg forward. The muscles at the back of the leg are relaxed. There is nothing to hinder the flow of his leg or stilt his action. Look at a tense person walking; they jerk along in a most ungainly way. The relaxed cat flows. When his leg moves backwards, the muscles at the back of the leg contract, those at the front relax.

I have seen many people take on a new grace and charm merely by learning to relax properly. Perhaps this was most marked in Edna, an elderly patient. As she learned to relax, the worry and tension left her face. Coupled with the benefits of the diet, a new vitality and vigour came over her, producing a genuine radiant glow that was obvious to all.

Very soon, using these techniques, your body will be relaxed, your mind also, and the benefits of the *meditation* will have entered your daily life. You will be reacting appropriately, and you will be heading towards maximum health.

Chapter five

POSITIVE THINKING

The power of the mind

Passive *meditation* produces its effects subtly. They flow on easily, automatically. We don't have to think of what we are doing; in fact the mind can stand in our way. To receive the benefits of this *meditation*, all we have to do is to practise the techniques and persevere.

However, the active mind does provide us with another vast – more concrete – resource. The power of the mind has the ability to create what we think. In doing so, it is very effective, but it does not discriminate. It will help us to success or failure, depending entirely upon the direction in which we channel it.

Studies in the United Kingdom have shown that cancer patients with a positive attitude, the will to live, do just that. They live longer than their pessimistic fellow-patients. More importantly, their quality of life is significantly better. It has been found that even the best treatment in the world is unlikely to work on a person with a negative outlook. The patient's attitudes are critical. I remember Anne, a lady who had been stable for a long time despite advanced cancer. Basically she was physically well, but she worried about her future and her children. She pestered her doctors to give an estimate of how long she would live. Repeatedly, she was told such crystal ball gazing was not possible. Then in a specialist's moment of exasperation with her, she was told, 'Three months'. Her husband told me that the effect was electric. Her condition began to deteriorate even before the consultation ended and she proved to be very punctual, dying exactly three months later.

Likewise, I remember my good friend who began intensive *meditation* with Dr Meares at the same time that I did. We were both enthusiastic about our prospects but both came to a crisis point at the same time. My crisis sent me off exploring a host of other avenues while she confided, 'I have tried everything else. I think Dr Meares has something. If he cannot save me, nothing can'. Totally committed, she battled on, passing through a very difficult time. Finally the crisis passed, her tumours subsided and she was in full remission. Her case was reported, the press congregated. However, all the attention unsettled her and she began to deteriorate. Withdrawing into relative seclusion and intensifying her efforts, she again picked up and remained well until Dr Meares went on a month's leave. By the time he returned, so had her tumours. Under his guidance and more intensive passive *meditation*, the cancer regressed again. Some months later, however, a friend pressured her to seek help from an alternative source. Although she was physically well and clear of tumours at the time, her mind was again thrown into disarray. Her resolve lost, my friend deteriorated rapidly and she died shortly afterwards. This is an incredible story of the *meditation's* ability to treat her cancer and of the ability of her active mind to undermine that effect.

Even more incredible is the story of an American hill-billy with throat cancer. Diagnosed by a local General Practitioner, he was told that he was being referred to the large city hospital to have a new form of ray treatment that would cure him. Arriving in awe at the hospital, he was given a basic check-up. When a thermometer was put in the naive man's mouth, his clinician was astute enough to realise that the hill-billy thought this was the new wonder treatment. After several sessions of this 'treatment', the cancer disappeared completely!

While we might smile at the mental picture of a simple hill-billy being cured by a thermometer, let us not lose sight of the importance of the principle he demonstrated so well. The message is that positive thinking works. What we need is a framework, acceptable to modern, critical man, upon which we can build that same positivity.

If we 'believe in' our specialist and he flatly states that we have three months to live, another great hurdle to getting well is created. On the other hand, I was particularly blessed in always having a very positive outlook. I felt sure that I would recover. I was doubly blessed by having Grace's support and equally optimistic approach. Even when I slid to within two weeks of what my doctor thought was imminent death, we both felt that we would find a solution. We did, of course, and I see this same positive attitude in all the people I have met who have similarly overcome their cancer. If they did not have it to begin with, they learned to develop their positivity.

This is the exciting thing – positivity can be learned! This is doubly important when we see how much it helps those around us. Being the centre of attention in this situation, if we are positive it rubs off on everyone else. So, if you go to your doctor and are optimistic and enthusiastic, he is likely to try that little bit harder to give a little more, and you get added benefit.

My friend Jazzer was the master at this. Having Hodgkins' Disease, he went through six years of treatment that caused him many problems. Whenever he went for more treatment, however, his natural inclination was to make the doctors and nurses feel good and to make the most of his situation. His infectious wit left a sea of smiling faces and the staff both loved him and did all they could for him. When he became resistant to the treatments available, he still had enough spark left to set off on his own search for health. Friends rallied to support him and, largely through healing and nutrition, he is in full remission – smiling more than ever!

So, having made that first basic decision that you do want to get better, you need positivity! If you have it already, count your blessings and see if you can make more of it. If you doubt its presence, or know it to be lacking, the first step is one of clear-cut choice. You are either positive or you are not. You must choose to be positive and then follow through the steps that develop it. This act of choice is a crucial one.

Do not pass it off as being too simplistic to just choose to be positive. It is that simple. This is one of those basic choices in life that should and can be made consciously. We must fix it in our minds to be positive. It must become a firm attitude that we hold and strengthen at every opportunity.

We can do this with the aid of active meditation and contemplation. This is another procedure which is very different to the basic, passive *meditation* we have learned already. To get the benefit here, we can actively meditate upon a particular topic – positivity!

To do this, take up your usual *meditation* position and get the body deeply relaxed as you would normally when using this technique. Then, instead of aiming for a still mind, you actively concentrate on what positivity means to you. You meditate upon the concept of positivity. You actively think about it, consider it from every viewpoint. You think of how you would define it, compare it with negativity, think of positive people you know, think of positive aspects of your own character. Think of why you want to be more positive.

As you meditate on it more, you will get a very comprehensive feeling about positivity and what it means to you. This may take one or more sessions. Do this regularly until you feel that you have achieved an overview of it all. You will then be contemplating 'positivity' and new insights may come.

Now make a decision. Say to yourself, 'I am a positive person now'. Repeat this affirmation over and over to yourself, until you know it carries conviction. Affirmations are wonderful things. They work! By using such simple, positive statements and repeating them regularly, we can condition our thoughts so that they lead on to the actions we intend.

So, when you first get up in the morning, repeat to yourself, 'I am a positive person now', for two minutes. Make time to do it again at least twice more during the day. Especially when driving in the car, say it out loud – even sing it if you like! Again a sense of fun is good, so put it to different tunes, be theatrical, but keep doing it. Because then, when a decision needs to be made, you will have a little voice in the back of your mind saying, 'I am a positive person now'. And Bingo! You will make a positive decision! As you become more positive, you see the system work, and it becomes that much easier to be positive the next time. As the intended actions are put into practice, the cycle of positivity is completed and will then steadily help to build a better life.

You will soon find that you have a new feeling, a feeling of being responsible for your own situation. You will be doing everything because you feel positive about it. You want to do it; it is your choice. You will feel in control of your situation and you will find that your inner resources will be strengthening and developing rapidly.

You will come to recognise that if you were not positive before, you almost certainly suffered from 'victim consciousness'. This is the 'Why me?' syndrome, the attitude that leaves people feeling a powerless pawn of a random fate that has slated them for doom. It is the most negative and destructive attitude in which you could have allowed yourself to indulge. If you recognise it from your new vantage point of positivity, be gentle with yourself. You are a positive person now. Quietly remind yourself that is not the way you are now. Seek out how you can change those negative aspects and not repeat them again.

When you do act positively, congratulate yourself. Quietly, of course! But happily. Reaffirm your new attitude and seek the next opportunity to practise it. You can reasonably expect to have ups and downs, so you must be prepared to *persevere*. That is the key to ultimate success. Once you have established it, there are some very important techniques for developing the basic urge to be positive.

Decision-making is a vital skill. You need to be sure and confident in all you do. There is a process available which will ensure you make decisions and make them positively. This process is summarised later. The decision to be made is first identified. Don't overlook this seemingly basic step. Knowing what needs to be done is a skill in itself.

So let us use the example of deciding what food to eat. You want to decide what is best for you to eat. The next step then is to collect information. With this example, the available information is vast and we could probably collect information forever. So we need to *set a time limit* – a time when the decision will be made. With food, we may choose a week to gather resources; with a simpler decision a day or an hour may be enough. Then, we *collect* as much *information* as possible from whatever sources we deem appropriate. Come the time for a decision, we need to *weigh up* the information. It may be helpful to write down the points for and against the various possibilities. While the rational, left side of the brain must play a big role, don't forget the other half, the intuitive half. I strongly recommend that in major decisions you also use the technique of *contemplation*.

To do this, relax first, then concentrate on all aspects of the impending decision, then meditate and contemplate. By doing so you will develop a profound understanding of the issues and may well gain new insights into any problem areas. Then you can feel far more positive about your final decision. Likewise, give credence to your intuition, which often expresses itself during contemplation. Whatever process you use, however, you must then come to a *decision*. Some people find decisions easy to make, others hard. If you find it hard to begin with, this process should soon help. If all else fails, toss a coin! But do make your decisions in a clearcut way.

Now, the vital step: *Accept* that this is the best decision you can make in the circumstances. You must be prepared to accept it fully. Some decisions will have both advantages and disadvantages and are taken because on balance they seem to offer the best prospects. You must be able to accept this wisdom and assure yourself that, given the present situation and facts, this decision is the best one to follow. Then you must be prepared to make light of any drawbacks and concentrate on *making your decision work to the fullest.*

This resolve may be strengthened by using affirmations or visualisation. *Affirmations* are truly wonderful as, when you begin to use them, it does not matter if you believe what you are repeating, or not. Keep repeating an affirmation and it will happen.

While writing this book I took some time in exile away from the family to concentrate on finishing it. Although tired to begin with, I affirmed, 'I have an infinite supply of harmonious energy'. I began writing at 6 p.m., working continuously until 1.30 a.m. I was able to begin again at 8.30 a.m. next morning, working solidly until 1 a.m. the next morning with only a few short breaks.

Affirmations are excellent aids to changing old patterns. If you decide you would like to do something differently, react in a better way, whatever, try affirmations. By making a clear, accurate statement of what you need to happen and repeating it, you will automatically begin to make the right decisions to effect it. Don't be sceptical about this. It is not false imagining; affirmations do work. The only effort is in needing something enough to get a clear picture of what it is that you really need. Then you must ask for it, clearly and precisely. If it is working well you only have to ask once. I know if I go shopping in the city and ask for a parking space outside any busy store, it will be there. I have done it for years.

However, if by chance I forget to mentally ask, it is never there! Understandably, parking spaces are important to me, but I am also confident that the process will work with all else. Nevertheless, there are things for which I will not ask. Perhaps this is a left-over from old conditioning; perhaps an acceptance of personal limitations, but my confidence remains and I *know* the basic process works. I also know my *wants* are different to my *needs*. Often there are things that I may want, but not necessarily need! If you really need something, ask and you shall receive. Just be sure you really need it; then you can be certain that it will arrive.

Visualisation works in the same way. Instead of stating your intentions, you *see* them in your mind. So, see yourself doing positive things, driving into the required parking space, eating the right food, getting well again, being joyful. You could finish your passive *meditation* by visualising yourself whole and healthy running along the beach. The frequent use of such images of health and happiness is very valuable.

In the United States, a radiologist and his psychologist wife have combined relaxation with visualisation to harness this healing potential in a very specific way. In their excellent book *Getting Well Again* the Simontons describe how they train people to use their minds to actively do battle with the cancer.[3] Their techniques undoubtedly bring results and are worth considering. These techniques are used in conjunction with radiation and they certainly can be used also by people having chemotherapy.

The starting point is physical relaxation. Then with eyes closed, a mental image is built up which involves the cancer cells being weak and confused. The treatment is seen to be strong and powerful and destroying the cancer cells. The healthy tissues around the diseased ones are seen as having no trouble in recovering from any damage the treatment might cause. The body's own defence system, through the white blood cells, then swarms in to mop up the remnants of the cancer cells. This removes the cancer entirely from the body. Finally, the patients see themselves in total health, fulfilling their goals in life.

The Simontons encourage patients to do this imaging in symbolic terms. So the cancer cells may be seen as minced steak, the white blood cells as dogs running in to eat it up. This preserves a non-literal, symbolic quality which most people find easier to do.

I did have some chemotherapy and during it I used these techniques – or rather, a variation of them as at that time I had not heard of Simontons. When I was actually having the drugs run-in, I relaxed as thoroughly as I could. With my eyes closed, I would welcome the drugs and visualise them going to the site of my cancer and killing the diseased cells there. Having a reasonable knowledge of the cell types involved, I actually visualised my bone cancer cells being destroyed. Then I visualised other, specialised cells that came in and ate up this excess bone that my cancer had formed. These osteoclasts, as they are called, are normally active in the process of bone remodelling and reshaping, and I am sure this visualisation helped my chest return to normal. For me, it was a simple image, and one with which I felt both comfortable and confident. I used the technique frequently.

However, the method is not without its problems. For patients who do develop a strong, effective image the results can be very good. If, on the other hand, there is doubt or, worse, a deep sense that the treatment will not work, these techniques could reinforce these fears, thus strengthening the cancer itself and so making it more resistant to treatment. Having seen one instance of this occurring I am cautious. There was a lady in our group who had stabilised her cancer, using nothing but diet and meditation. It stayed stable for eighteen months, but she grew impatient when it did not go away completely. She still had a fear that her active cancer state would recur. She began to use this visualisation technique on her own and, as it turned out, her images were not completely positive. A short time later the cancer did reappear and she felt compelled to accept standard treatments.

I believe visualisation to be a good technique, but one that requires close co-operation and monitoring from someone fully versed in it. For this reason, I have not talked of it much in public. Also, it is my personal view that the symbols used in visualisations should not be aggressive. Dogs tearing at meat or opposing armies doing battle are images of conflict which I would not choose. To work with my body I prefer to maintain a sense of co-operation and respect. Even when using this technique in association with treatments such as chemotherapy or radiation, which are basically aggressive and destructive, I feel more at ease with those natural, co-operative images which are discussed a little further on in this chapter.

The other concern I have about visualisation is that nature did not intend the mind to be *consciously* involved in the details of a healing process. Our automatic, self-healing processes work well once the right conditions are created and we do not need to dwell on them *in detail*. Imagine trying to dictate to your body the steps it should take in repairing a broken leg. You would need detailed pathological knowledge to even begin, and the chance of visualising all the complex sequence of events in their correct order would be still slim.

We can, however, use our mind to help create the ideal conditions in which healing can proceed. By repeatedly forming images of health and wholeness in our mind, we can programme ourselves to achieve just that. This is particularly helpful in the cancer situation when we are likely to be faced with so many negative images. Whether it be our own poor expectations, the careless remarks of medical personnel or thoughtlessness of friends and relations, this negative input needs to be counter-balanced with images of healing and health.

Visualisation works very well towards creating a positive personal image. As I prefer peace to conflict, I prefer to use images of co-operation involving the body simply doing what it was intended to do, that is returning itself to health. This is why I did a fairly 'literal' form of visualisation when having chemotherapy and why I used the radiant light technique described earlier.

It is fine, however, to visualise the external treatments of chemotherapy or radiation destroying cancer cells. If you have chosen to use these treatments, that is what you want them to do. At the same time, however, visualise the rest of the body being strong and healthy and becoming more so, and *see it* being unaffected by the treatment. In this way you are actually working with the treatment to make it more effective.

This can be done in the way that I did it by learning about the actual processes involved and visualising them in your mind. Alternatively, it can be done abstractly in the way discussed by the Simontons; that is using symbols for the treatment, the cancer, the body's defences and your own resulting good health.

If you choose to use symbols, then first sit quietly and relax physically. Next, think of an image – a symbol for each of the components in the process you are seeking to enhance. Look for related symbols that naturally evoke the effect you are seeking. The resulting images and the loadings individuals put on them vary so much from person to person that it would be unwise of me to attempt to describe an 'ideal' set of symbols. Everyone will produce something different. The challenge is to be sure that it is a positive image *for you.*

For example, Geoff visualised his cancer as a snowball rolling downhill and his own defences being the sun melting it away. My conception of snowballs rolling downhill is that they get bigger and bigger as they go! So, while it might be fine for him, this image would not work for me. Again I stress – if in doubt, seek professional guidance.

A third, much safer way of visualising can be applicable to all situations. This is an even more abstract and harmonious form which relies on powerful symbols. Also, we have talked of using the image of running along the beach.

The radiant light is one example. Dr Alec Forbes at the Bristol Cancer Care Centre has used another more involved sequence. This begins with relaxing physically then embarking on an imaginary, inwardly visualised journey. This journey puts together a number of archetypal symbols as used by Carl Jung and later employed in psychosynthesis. It is a very pleasant way of creating a healthy, positive and integrated self-image.

Again, it begins with sitting comfortably and going through the relaxation exercise. Then, with your eyes closed, you imagine going into a field. It is 'your' field, a place which you know for its 'specialness'. It may be an actual field, or a product of your imagination. You walk across it, gazing at its beauty. You feel the grass beneath your feet, and the warm breeze on your face. You can hear the pleasant sounds of birds and crickets and the wind sighing in the trees. You smell the sweet smells of the pasture.

You come to a pool in the field which can be deep or shallow, depending on whether you are a swimmer or a paddler. You take off your clothes and, leaving your troubles with them on the bank, you enter the water to enjoy yourself. If you want to wash, then wash; if you want to swim, then swim. You may care to drink some of the sweet water. After a while you come out on to the opposite bank where there is a waterfall. You shower in the waterfall, then pass through it to a cave behind. The entrance to the cave is lit by shimmering light from the waterfall and as you walk into the cave you see a bright light at the other end. It is sunlight. As you come out of the cave you find yourself in a pleasant glade. There are flowers and trees and shrubs and as you walk on you come to a bench with towels and new, clean clothes. You dry yourself and put on the clothes and then walk back through a wood to your field – to where you began.

Either of these visualisations, the 'radiant light' or the 'inward journey', is excellent to use at the end of passive *meditation*. It is also suitable to do active imagery, using the Simontons' principles, after *meditation* for then you are combining the benefits of the processes of mind-stilling and mind-sharpening.

Summary of visualisation

Both the Simontons' and Forbes' techniques can be useful. The Simontons' method is particularly useful if chemotherapy or radiation is being used. Their work shows it is likely to increase the treatment's effect dramatically as well as increasing the patient's level of co-operation and well-being. Dr Forbes' 'journey' is helpful for all.

My attitude is that these things can be useful extras to add once the passive *meditation* is working for you. Because they are active, mind techniques, they do not provide the Release that *meditation* does, but they do help in other ways. So get the *meditation* working well first. Be aware of your time commitments and priorities and, if you feel you wish to try these extra techniques, then do so. Make sure your images *are* positive ones and if there is the slightest doubt, seek suitable help with them. Remember:

1 The mind certainly can work for us, but it needs to be directed appropriately.

2 In cancer, the patient's belief systems and level of well-being can make all the difference between success and failure.

3 A happy person heals rapidly, an unhappy one slowly.

4 We do not necessarily need to think actively of the healing process to affect it, but an overall positive attitude is a great asset.

5 To repeat, the body heals itself automatically once the right conditions are provided.

6 The mind, however, can have a great influence on those conditions and the healing process itself.

7 It is appropriate to use mind-stilling and mind-sharpening techniques.

Whether you use affirmation and visualisation techniques or not, when making decisions work positively you obviously must act according to those decisions. There is the obvious danger of not following through with a good idea. It is so *easy* to be enthused and filled with resolve one day, only to be lured in other directions the next. Do not allow those excuses that seem so real prevent you taking the action you had intended. Accept that there will be hurdles to overcome. You will have good days and bad days. The final quality required in developing positivity is *perseverance*. You must keep on until your goals are reached.

Perseverance takes *discipline* and this can also be developed. It is very worthwhile to practise also. Do something each day purely as an exercise in discipline. Perhaps go without a piece of food you would have had for pleasure's sake; do exercises as an act of discipline; even do as I do – finish your daily shower by turning the hot tap off and the cold full on. This for me takes great discipline! Although it is extremely invigorating and I have been doing it for years, it still takes effort for me to do it. Practising discipline by choice makes it a little easier to use self-discipline where more important – such as persevering through the ups and downs of the healing process. If you use this decision-making process you will make the right decisions for your situation. If you act on those decisions and persevere, you will achieve your goals.

So using food as an example of how to approach the decision-making process, you weigh the possibilities and decide the maintenance diet which suits you best and then embrace it fully. If you have been used to cooking with salt and find food bland without it, look for new flavours. You will soon find that your sense of taste improves remarkably, and all the vegetables that once tasted the same do in fact have very pleasant individual characters. You could affirm, 'I am sensitive to the appropriate food to maximise my health'. You could visualise yourself with good appetite, eating and enjoying the food you feel appropriate to your situation.

You may like to set yourself a time to try the new decision. With a new way of eating we may give ourselves one month. So, for the next month, it is maintenance diet one hundred per cent. Resist wavering, or thinking about adding this or that during this time. You have made a decision and set a goal to try it for one month. Do it fully. At the end of that month, reassess the situation. Has the decision worked as you planned? Do you need to modify it? If the plan has had shortcomings, and you have given it a maximum trial, you will have no nagging doubts that begin with, 'I wonder whether it would have worked better if . . .?' You will be content to leave that line and try something else. If it has been all you hoped for and you see the benefits, you will feel more confident to take the next step. Set another time goal and follow through, reassessing at the end of the period. Be sensitive to what agrees with you and what does not. As you do this more and more, your confidence will grow and you will steadily build up your health.

The next part of the positive approach is to work at creating what we call a <u>healing environment</u>. These are all the little things, some quite subtle, which go further towards creating that ideal environment in which your body can proceed towards health.

You can reinforce your confidence and positivity through the examples of others. Avoid negative pessimists and seek out the company of bright people who make you feel good. If necessary, tactfully ask those people you wish to avoid to stay away until you feel stronger. There was one lady, Shirley, who, when low, felt physically assaulted by a very intrusive, gossiping friend. She was friend enough, however, to respect the request not to call for a time, and the friendship resumed after a regenerating interlude.

A group of people doing the same thing provides great moral support. We find that new people joining our groups are lifted by the positive attitudes of those who are already practising the techniques. Seeing newcomers lifted to a better quality of life reinforces the older member's confidence, and so the group's positivity steadily builds. You can be the agent to catalyse this same effect in your own community if you want to. Seek out ways in which you can make other people happy. Take the initiative. Tell your visitors how well they look, how pleased you are to see them. Find the way to make their day happier, and everyone will benefit.

Once you begin you will find there are many ways to increase your momentum. In sorting priorities, the value of verbalising needs to be emphasised. Either writing of, or talking about your problems gives a broader perspective, lightens your load and produces better results.

Keeping a daily diary is a very valuable habit. I used an exercise book and wrote regularly on what I had done and what I was planning. To write like that requires clarifying the issues in your mind and so aids the decision-making and assessing process. Also, I found it helpful to be able to go back over what I had written months before and assess my progress. Particularly when passing through a flat patch, this can be very reassuring.

Similarly, it is desirable to cultivate someone with whom you can talk – someone with whom you can really discuss things openly and honestly, on a heart-to-heart level.

You may need to seek out such a person. If you feel comfortable doing this with a relative, it works well, but frequently people feel more at ease with a friend, or even someone removed from the situation. If you would like to cultivate a friend, then do just that. Actually ask them if they are prepared to be your listening post when you need someone to talk to. Anyone would be flattered to be asked such a thing. If there is no one close by to fill this role, then seek out the professional help of a medical person, clergyman or trained counsellor. The benefits make it well worthwhile. You will find by talking to someone about your problems you will release any hold such difficulties have or tension they are causing. Often, if a problem seems insoluble, just talking about it will provide the new perspective that makes the answer obvious. Similarly, letter-writing can be a great means of communicating and sharing your experiences. As you send letters off and receive replies, a positive momentum is gained. Some people even find it helpful to write to members of their immediate family. By doing so they find it easier to share their thoughts and feelings and so maintain and develop their family ties.

In your personal relationships, honesty is essential. Consider that often-asked question, 'How are you today, dear?' Ugh! you think to yourself, I feel terrible, but no one's going to know! So you reply in a half-hearted way, 'Oh, I'm fine, thanks'. Rubbish! You know you are putting on a false front, and so does your friend.

Your dishonesty has created a barrier that not only will prevent other people from talking to you in the normal way they would, it has also reinforced the idea that cancer is a bogey that should be shunned.

Be positive. 'Well, I feel bloody terrible today, but I am doing this and that and tomorrow I expect to be feeling a lot better.' Immediately the atmosphere is different. You have respected your friend enough to tell them the truth. They will appreciate that, and if they want to talk more of your situation and make suggestions, then the way is open. You have made a positive statement and shown that you feel confident. Once your health has been discussed, you will be free to talk openly as you normally would on any subject.

Cancer can be overcome. Fear is one of cancer's greatest strengths. We, as cancer patients, can and should help the community to be free of that fear and so deal with it appropriately and successfully.

Reading adds to your positivity. There exists a wealth of inspirational and informative books from which to choose and they can reinforce you constantly. [See References and Further Reading listed at the end of this book.] We were amazed at how often reading solved our problems as we searched for the right answer to health. Often we were confronted by a situation for which we knew no solution. Regularly, the next book we were drawn to read contained the answer! As we became aware of this, we found we often just 'felt our way' to a particular book and that it 'fell open' at the page with the answer.

Having experienced this so often, I do not decry intuition – or whatever else it may be called. The more we accepted it, the better it worked. A friend had a particularly graphic example of how 'coincidences' can be so meaningful. John was a multiple sclerosis patient who had been severely handicapped and now was working his way steadily back to health. He reached an impasse at a particular point, however, and was feeling desperate. One morning he went out to collect his newspaper. Not only had the wrong one been delivered to his box, a most unusual happening – but the wind had blown it out of the box, scattering it against his door. As he leaned down to pick it up a name leapt from the print and caught his attention. It was the name of an old dear friend, in the death notices. John attended the funeral and afterwards, feeling rather melancholic, browsed through a bookshop. Walking down the rows of books, one book was hanging half-way out of the case. Glancing at the title, John was staggered. His friend's name, Christian and surname, was on the cover! Not written by his friend, but by another of the same name, this book was devoted to the topic besetting him! We last heard of John full of excitement after returning from a five-mile bush walk, an impossibility for him to even consider a year previously.

I feel it wise to be sensitive to your intuition and be prepared for hints to your direction. We found that the best avenues to follow were the ones that flowed smoothly. Those surrounded by difficulty were usually dead-ends. This special direction we acquired made us more positive each time we experienced it. We no longer believe in 'coincidences'.

Your state of mind will also benefit from good, old-fashioned, regular physical exercise. This will do more than merely aid your body to relax and give it greater vitality. You will find it beneficial emotionally and mentally. The American Heart Foundation recommends that one hour of formal exercise three times each week is enough to provide the basic level of benefit. They say that you should choose a form of exercise appropriate to your situation. For those in bed, a series of arm exercises may be enough. For the most adventurous, jogging or more strenuous exercise will be appropriate. Remember that you need to work within your limits. One of the best guides as to your personal acceptable limit to exercise is that if you overdo it, and so stress your heart, you will be unable to keep up a conversation. So, if you do go jogging and you get to the point where you cannot talk easily, slow to a walk until you can, then recommence. It is best to take it quietly to begin with.

Many people choose to exercise daily, particularly as they notice the benefits they derive from it. Walking is the most common form of exercise for older people, and many make a half-hour walk after dinner a regular part of the day. We have bike riders, tennis players, swimmers, and people following programmes of regular gym exercises in our groups. They look fitter and healthier than most people you meet in the street. One man complained in a laughing way about looking so well. 'I am meant to be so ill, yet I look so good, I cannot even get any sympathy!' He continues to look well.

I also gained greatly from practising breathing exercises and recommend them highly. A short session first thing in the morning, outside in the fresh air, preferably with bare feet in contact with the earth and certainly the eyes free of glasses, is a great start to any day.

The best breathing exercises have their origin in Yoga. Called Pranayama in India, they are intended to purify the blood, nerves and lungs, and to be an aid in developing mental concentration and stability.[4] Noble aims, indeed, and another valuable tool we can use in our aim of maximising health. Most Yoga Schools concentrate heavily on breathing exercises. Ramacharaka's books are the best I know on the subject. [See Further Reading.]

It becomes obvious that our whole environment enhances the quality of our life and can be used to aid the healing process. The more harmony we seek and find, the better we feel and progress. We should take advantage of good, soothing music and colours. Avoid jingly-jangly, jarring effects and take a guide from nature. Trips into the countryside are well worthwhile, and there is more that we can do at home to absorb soothing rhythms and feel the true harmony of good living.

A creative activity is a must. Nothing feeds the soul like seeing something creative flow from our own hand. It bolsters our self-esteem and satisfies a basic aspect of our human nature. If you have ever painted, knitted, made furniture, clothes or whatever, rekindle the interest. If not, develop a new one! Gardening is an excellent outlet. It is wonderfully creative, it takes you into nature, you can grow your own food, and you can cultivate beauty in the form of glorious flowers, all while you get fresh air and exercise. It has a host of good features and is my favourite activity. While on the gardening theme, it is good to cultivate indoor plants. They bring nature inside, adding freshness and life to the healing environment.

Helping others is a great way to help yourself. Being a patient, it is often easy to feel everything should be done for you and you have a right to be self-centred. In fact, the more you give the more you receive, so look for ways of helping others. Many in our groups do voluntary work in hospitals or the community. Some just look for extra ways to help friends and family. Prayer offers a way that patients confined to bed can help others. In all these things people find that not only do they get more in return, but just the doing feels good.

And let us not forget laughter. Yes, laughter. With all there is to consider and do it would be easy to become so earnest and serious that we could overlook enjoying ourselves! Take time out to really laugh, it is a wonderful means of Release. Go to the comedy shows. Get the old-time Buster Keaton and Charlie Chaplin video tapes. Borrow books from the library's humour section and make the effort to laugh heartily. Be inspired by Norm Cousins' *Anatomy of an Illness* and learn how he used laughter as a primary aid to curing his chronic degenerative disease.[5]

Laughter is almost as important a tool as that most important one of all, *meditation* which, in its passive form, subtly and steadily builds a positive attitude. As you practise it you become unaffected by stress and anxiety. You will just simply feel good. You feel like doing the right thing. You become more likely to make the right decisions.

Cancer patients often come to us feeling there is nothing they can do to help themselves. Soon they have so many decisions to make, so many things to consider as aids to getting well again. Where is the time for it all? What are the priorities? Perhaps then is the time to recall the beautiful Chinese maxim: 'The journey of a thousand miles begins with just one step.'

I would consider *meditation* as the ideal first step. Do it first, and do it well. If you find that completely satisfying, it could be enough. I imagine, however, that you will feel the need to consider your dietary situation and that also there will be many other things to consider. Use the decision-making techniques to decide your priorities and plan a course of action. Consider the many possibilities, and add what you feel appropriate for yourself at this particular time. There will probably be one or two things mentioned that seem to leap off the page at you. Some of the ideas mentioned, you may well be utilising already; others you may want to use later. Start with what seems particularly relevant and important for you.

Meditation, diet and positive thinking are the pillars on which to build. You can use any number of other aids as the bricks with which to complete the final edifice of health. This, then, is a summary of the possible ways of creating and maintaining a positive attitude.

1 Positive thinking
 Choose to be positive
 Meditate and contemplate it
 Decide to do it
 Affirm it, visualise yourself doing it
 Practise it
 Persevere

2 The decision-making process
 Identify the decision to be made
 Set a time when the decision will be made
 Collect information, record it if necessary
 Contemplate
 Assess
 Decide
 Accept your decision as the best one you can make in the circumstances
 Aim to maximise benefits, minimise drawbacks
 Set goals (may include trial period)
 Act according to decision – commit yourself
 Reinforce with visualisation or affirmations, if necessary
 Re-assess regularly
 Persevere
 Discipline

3 Creating the healing environment
 Inspiration
 Diet
 Verbalise
 ● diary
 ● cultivated listener
 ● develop communication skills
 ● letter writing
 Reading
 Exercise
 ● physical
 ● breathing

Music, colour, nature, atmosphere
Creative activity
Laughter
Help others
Active visualisation
● literal images
● symbolic images used in association with treatment
● abstract images used in all contexts
Passive *meditation*

As I was working back to health, Grace and I aimed, at every stage, to concentrate on one thing at a time. When that had been explored and assessed, we either integrated it into our programme or happily left it out. Adjustments were constantly made – still are being made – as we seek our optimum. We now encourage others to do likewise. It is a gradual, cumulative process which aims to build towards total health.

Be sensitive to your own physical and psychological limits. It is impossible to do it all today, or even by tomorrow! It takes time. This was a hard one for me to learn. Having been used to training hard in athletics for the Decathlon, I found it difficult to adjust to new limitations. In the early days I landed in quite deep water by over-taxing myself physically and trying to do too much. Even in the last few years there have been times when my body has warned me to take time off, to indulge in a change of pace with a holiday and some recreation.

Learning to keep within your own physical and psychological limits is a necessary art to acquire. The challenge is to work towards that combination of things that will produce the best results for you, as an individual, in terms of quality of life and quantity of life.

Decide your priorities first. Making a written list of them is a great help. Then you will need the discipline to follow through on your decisions and to carry out your plan for health. Be assured that others have done it already, while more are doing it now. They became, invariably, 'weller than well'.

Chapter six

PAIN CONTROL

It's only pain!

We have talked of fear being a basic hurdle to overcome in the process of getting well again. Cancer is associated with two main fears: the fear that it will cause pain and the fear that it will lead to death. These fears are the primary reason why society dreads hearing or relating to the word 'cancer'; pain and death being the two things that our community has chosen to avoid at all costs. We have trained a culture that regards them with horror and treats them as unmanageable, negative events. As a result, they are often approached with a sense of panic as the individual feels powerless to help himself through the situation. This often leads people to rely on external aids which often do nothing for their quality of life.

The influence of fear extends beyond the patients themselves, as often relatives and friends become preoccupied with whether their loved ones are 'in pain' or not. This concern is natural and reasonable, but in my experience, usually accentuated and often clouded by the relatives' own personal fears. This leads to an unnatural preoccupation and is frequently a cause for tension and anxiety which in turn prevents dealing with problems on a more satisfactory level. Pain should be controlled, but total quality of life remains of paramount importance. There is no answer in being a society of pill-poppers rushing for the analgesics at the slightest twinge.

What is needed is a fresh approach that develops the individual's ability to manage most, if not all, of the pain that may come their way. Of course, you do not need to be a cancer patient to derive benefit from such an approach. I see this as a fundamental prerequisite in self-defence. If pain could be handled without fear or difficulty, it would be a great thing.

There is such a concept. It makes the self-management of pain a very real possibility, but it involves a technique that is totally new to most people.

Before discussing pain control further, it is well to extend a warning. *Pain is a signal that something is wrong.* It is important to know just what is wrong, to heed any warnings and to take such appropriate action as is necessary. People can learn to be unaffected by pain so that headaches do not bother them, so that back pain does not inconvenience their movement. That is fine if the pain is chronic and the person can be sure that it does not indicate a need for other or more treatment. Anne had three collapsed vertebrae in her spine. She used these methods to such effect that all the initially excruciating pain was gone and her mobility returned to normal. She then had to be extremely careful not to overdo her exercise as her back was very unstable. Similarly, it is important to know, before you turn a headache off, that it is just a simple headache and does not have a more serious cause.

So, having established that pain has its purpose, the basic premise we work with is that true pain does not hurt! You will come to see that this apparently extravagant claim is true. To begin with, however, it may be well removed from your normal experience of pain. We all know from past experience that when we feel a pain which goes beyond a certain level it jolly well hurts. Whether the pain is coming from a physical cause, such as a cut finger, or a psychological cause such as a broken romance, if we feel pain we normally expect it to hurt.

There is no doubt that if you do feel pain and it persists, then that pain can easily consume your interest and demand your attention. Everything else rapidly becomes secondary to it. If pain is a reality for you, its treatment requires top priority.

So, having said that we normally experience pain as hurting, and having myself had what is reputedly one of the most painful types of cancer, how can I say that true pain does not hurt? *True* pain does not hurt. Not many people have experienced true pain. Once we do understand the nature of pain and its basic components we can come to experience it ourselves, and learn that pain does not have to hurt.

Pain is a stimulus which we regard as unpleasant and which acts as a warning signal. It is an indication that something is wrong.

We need to appreciate that the something wrong can be of a physical, psychological or even spiritual nature. Commonly we regard pain as a purely physical event and this is why we have so much trouble dealing with it appropriately. Purely physical pain is what I call true pain and it does not hurt. We humans rarely feel such pain as most of our pain is coloured by psychological overtones. Animals, on the other hand, ably demonstrate the nature of true, physical pain.

I recall a little puppy that came into the surgery not so long ago. It was four months old and owned by a policeman. He rushed into the surgery with it, saying that it had been hit by a car and he thought he ought to shoot it, but first he wondered if we could do anything.

When I first saw the puppy I could not imagine what the problem was because all I could see was a little puppy looking around the surgery with a smile on its face and wagging its tail. It reacted just like any exuberant little puppy would, trying to give me a lick and wagging its tail. When I looked at its front legs, however, I found all the skin had been stripped right off them and both wrists were broken. The two open joints were just hanging loose. I am sure that, for a human, the shock alone would have put them in a very precarious position, but here was this little puppy looking around the surgery as if nothing had happened.

When I went to examine him and had to move his legs, his initial response was to try and pull out of the way. When he could not get away from me he tried to nip me. Not very seriously, but he was definitely trying to tell me that he'd rather I didn't do what I was trying to do. So the nurse held his head. Now he couldn't get out of the way and couldn't bite us, he immediately accepted his position and allowed us to examine him. His tail stopped wagging and he looked a bit unhappy about it all, but soon we had finished looking at his legs and put them back down on the table. His tail started wagging again and he went back to looking round the room as if nothing had happened.

Later we gave him an anaesthetic to clean him up as best we could and to keep his legs still while the plaster casts we used set hard. About two months later the casts came off and that little puppy was walking around again. Over the next month all the hair grew back on his legs. He was a normal dog again!

To me, that experience really shows up what is involved with pain and how to deal with it. It was a remarkable demonstration of how pain in its proper context does not hurt. Pain is a stimulus. For the puppy, his pain was a warning signal. It told him that if he moved, or was moved, his legs hurt more. He did all he could to remain still. He made the appropriate response to the stimulus. If he had been in the wild, and could have kept still long enough, his legs may well have healed just as they did in our plaster casts.

The pain was a warning stimulus; not pleasant, presumably, but still for the puppy, only a stimulus. When he was in a position of minimal discomfort, he was quite ready to accept that stimulus and make the most of his situation.

Contrast the puppy's reaction with our own on breaking a leg. We would have the initial physical pain of the event that caused the break. But in the same instant of such an accident our mind starts to race. 'Hell, I've broken my leg! Will I ever walk again? Is my insurance up to date? Who's going to do my work for me? How will I pay the bills while I'm in hospital?' And on and on it goes. This is the psychological aspect of pain. The worry and anxiety; the fear that goes with it.

True physical pain does not hurt. It is merely an unpleasant stimulus. Psychological pain can be excruciatingly hurtful. Understanding the difference between the physical and psychological aspects of pain is fundamental to dealing with it in the most appropriate manner.

Consider a day of 42 degrees Celsius. Hot, uncomfortable – but painful? Very few people would consider it to be so. We know the pure physical effect of such a temperature is not likely to be harmful and, anyway, it will probably be cooler tommorow. We tolerate it and go on with our business as best we can.

Yet imagine what would happen if people started dying when the temperature reached 43 degrees Celsius! The psychological component of pain would swing into action. Faced with a reason to fear the temperature, people would no doubt become preoccupied with the weather and limit their activities dramatically. I am sure that as a consequence 42 degrees Celsius would suddenly become a very painful temperature indeed!

This psychological component of pain is so strong in humans. Surely it accounts for that wonderful phenomenon, the placebo effect. A placebo is a blank pill, usually made of sugar, that is used to test the effectiveness of active drugs for a given condition. Many trials have shown the effectiveness of placebos in controlling even the most severe pain and there is ample medical evidence of their dramatic effects in many conditions. For more details, refer to N. Cousins' *Anatomy of an Illness.*[6]

We need to appreciate what the placebo is demonstrating. If a sugar pill can relieve pain for us, surely we can learn to do it for ourselves and derive the satisfaction that we otherwise laughingly bestow on the placebo.

A placebo is an external agent which we can accept as a treatment for the non-physical aspect of our condition. We can learn to harness the placebo effect and put it to work for ourselves.

We can experience pain in its true, pure, non-hurtful and manageable form. This, to me, is a basic technique in self-defence that everyone should know. Through it we can become free of the fear of pain and improve our level of well-being enormously.

I used to have a very low pain threshold. In my athletic days, when I was fit I could run a reasonable four hundred metres, but my performance was poor at any further distance. It hurt too much! To run a fast mile, or especially something like a marathon, you require a very high pain threshold indeed. I could not handle it. In the past, even just having stitches taken out was for me an acutely painful experience. I remember when my leg was amputated, however, that I avoided analgesics wherever possible. I was afraid I might become conditioned to them. The bone cancer I had is normally very painful and, not knowing any better then, I was quite afraid. If the cancer recurred, what would I do if the analgesics did not work? How could I handle chronic, severe pain?

I learned through experience and by training in pain! Seriously, we train in so many things to increase our ability in that area. In athletics I used to train hard to improve my performance. No one would consider that strange. Why not train ourselves to better our performance in dealing with pain?

By doing so myself, I have freed a whole area of my life. I no longer have fear of pain. Whereas before I used to be scared stiff of visits to the dentist, now I see it as an opportunity to confirm my freedom from the stranglehold pain held me in. I have been able to suture my own cuts without anaesthetic and again marvel at how pain, true pain, really does not hurt.

I have seen others benefit, too. I remember a young man, John, who had a deep fear of the pain of injections. Being on chemotherapy, his fear caused great difficulties. Each time he was to be injected, he would reflexly pull his arm away with a rapid jerk. Often it took eight or ten attempts to get the needle into his vein, causing anguish to all around.

After learning to relax and to cope with pain appropriately, he told me that not only did he stop the jerking but he did not even feel the needle going in.

To handle pain appropriately, we need to consider the psychological and the physical aspects. The starting point is to understand and accept pain. We then need to experience pain in its pure, non-hurtful form, to confirm our new attitudes about it. I strongly recommend this to everyone. Do not leave it until you have a pain and need to do it – get in first, and learn that pain does not have to hurt.

Our attitude towards pain is critical. Remember that for years we have been conditioned by a pain-fearing society to believe that pain hurts and should be avoided wherever possible. No doubt the real starting point lies in educating children to have a reasonable approach to it.

Pain should be approached in a non-emotional way. There is no need to make a fuss about it. If a child falls over and cuts itself, then comfort and treatment may well be required. There is no need to over-react, however. Children are conditioned by the emotions of those around them so quickly. Just watch the influence of a group of adults reacting to a small child's fall. 'Oh, my goodness!' they cry, as the hands fly up in horror. 'You poor thing, where does it hurt?'

We have seen society's effects on our own children. The eldest, Rosemary, initially had a remarkable pain tolerance. The normal bumps and scrapes she went through were only an annoyance to her. She was far more interested in getting back to learning, experiencing and doing to worry about pain. Up she would get and carry on, as Grace and I struggled to contain our own anxieties. Reinforced by her obvious lack of hurt, we were soon able to react in an appropriate way and the everyday minor accidents became non-events. After turning two, however, it took only a couple of episodes with doting elders gushing over some minor falls for her to begin reacting in the stereotyped way. Soon these same falls became a cause for tears and apparently genuine hurt. Interestingly, however, the worse the accidents, the less the reaction. Now it was as if the minor incidents were an outlet for pent-up emotions. It has taken several years to retrain her to accept pain and deal with it appropriately.

Not long ago Rosemary had a papilloma deep in her foot. It was quite irritating for her. Finally, being used to watching me work in the surgery, she declared she was going to cut it out. Didn't she think that would hurt? 'No, Daddy. I'll just make myself all floppy.' We had taught her how to relax herself and she is an expert at it. If she 'made herself all floppy' – deeply relaxed so her muscles were loose like a rag doll – she would not feel hurt. Relaxing herself thoroughly, she proceeded to take to the papilloma with some surgical scissors and excised it completely. The hardest thing was for Grace and I to control our reactions. Surely this was a reasonable thing to do with the annoyance, and it should be that easy. Perhaps we should not be surprised to see the theory at work. She can now deal with real pain well, but if emotionally agitated, the slightest accident produces a major outburst. She feels very little physical pain, but reacts strongly to psychological pain.

So the starting point in pain control is understanding and dealing with the psychological loadings we put on it. These loadings are basically either the product of fears or attempts at self-gain through pain.

The fears are easier to understand. They can be personal fears such as: Why am I hurting? Is it going to get worse? Will I recover? Am I going to die? They can be financial fears: Can I pay my medical bills? Will I be able to work again? Will I get my job back? They can be social ones: Will I be rejected? What will my family do? What will my friends think? Am I to be an outcast? It does not take long to run up a list of horrors that are all too real in any disease, and in cancer especially.

Perhaps the greatest need in dealing with such fears is being able to accept our situation as it is. If we can do that, and through acceptance deal with things as best we can, while at the same time avoiding worrying about what tomorrow may or may not bring, then we will be free from psychological pain. The 'if' that begins that last sentence may seem like a rather large one to begin with, but accepting our situation is something that can be done. Just realising the need to do it gets us halfway there. Then identifying what causes pain to hurt shows us how to deal with it. Regular *meditation* and positive thinking definitely lead to a peace of mind which engenders acceptance. Many people have found this and by using the techniques have come to experience a calmness that has been followed by an automatic lessening in their pain.

[Chapter 10 deals in much greater detail with how to tackle fears and replace them with positive emotions.]

The other side of our involvement with pain is the fact that often we have an ulterior motive in feeling pain. We are getting, or at least trying to get something, through the pain. This idea of pain having secondary gains for us is often a hard one to look at in your own life. It is almost certainly providing a greater or lesser component of any pain you might feel.

Many people feel guilty about being sick and so accept that they should be 'suffering'. To have cancer and be 'in pain' is all part of the expectation and punishment that such people accept. This self-image aspect is very important. Do you see yourself as a sick person going downhill, or do you regard yourself as temporarily ill and on the road to recovery? I am sure people in the latter group feel less hurt from the same stimulus.

Our personal reaction to pain is very much a product of our attitudes, emotional state and level of well-being. There is no need to punish ourselves by accepting pain. Again, use the positive thinking principles, giving close attention to concentrating on pleasant activities. Laughter beats aspirin any day!

Secondary gains also frequently involve the other people in our life. By being 'in pain', relatives and friends rally to us and often fill an emotional need we feel. Again, there is no need to feel guilty about realising this – unless you are doing it consciously! There has to be a better way. (See Chapter 10 for ways to fulfil your needs without indulging in sickness and pain.)

The psychological aspect of pain is, therefore, rather involved. To deal with it appropriately we need to understand our nature honestly and to look openly at what our goals are in life and how we want to achieve them. Again, this makes cancer an exercise in self-discovery and self-development.

As far as pain goes, understanding the psychological aspect gets us halfway to having it under control. To feel confident of being in control, however, we need to practise! Once we have experienced pure physical pain as a reality and know that it does not hurt, we can apply that knowledge to any experience of pain.

We can do this in a set exercise by detaching ourselves from the psychological aspect of pain and then applying a controlled painful stimulus. To avoid any psychological loadings, we need to feel secure, to be in control of the situation and divorced from the influence of our mind and emotions. We meet all these criteria admirably by doing the exercises initially while *meditating*.

We begin by choosing a suitable stimulus. We do not want to cause ourselves any bodily injury and so a paper clip of the 'bull-dog' type, works well. Remembering that everyone has a different pain threshold to begin with, find a convenient place on your arm or hand where the clip can be put to produce a tolerable stimulus. The upper part of the forearm has quite thick skin and is fairly tough. If the clip does not cause much reaction there, try the inner soft part of the arm. If need be, try the webbing between the fingers, or use just one corner of the clip. The aim is to produce a strong but acceptable stimulus. Putting it on ourselves leaves us in control. We know that we can stop the stimulus whenever we want to.

So, now take up your normal position for *meditation* and proceed to relax your body thoroughly. Let the mind come to rest also. Once settled, open your eyes a little, if necessary, and apply the clip. What reaction does it produce?

If you feel any hurt you will probably notice an automatic reflex. Your muscles will tense up. Probably those in the hand and arm will contract first; if you react a lot, the whole body may stiffen. Now, if you can impose relaxation on the body again, a strange thing happens. The hurt gradually goes away, leaving a pure stimulus. In the calm, you can experience true pain. The more you try this experiment, and become confident with it, the easier it is to experience true, non-hurtful pain.

The importance of this reflex is so useful to us, we must appreciate it fully. Not only does anxiety and stress lead to tension but, by doing so, it also leads on to hurtful pain. Similarly, relaxation relieves tension, defuses anxiety and stress, and takes the hurt out of pain. Relaxation is again the key. If we can keep our body relaxed, free of tension, we will find pain is well on the way to being controlled. This is why these exercises are easier and most effective if they are done while you are also practising *meditation* each day in the standard simple way.

Following these early, easy experiments, we need then to go on to bigger and better things. Increase the level of stimulus first by using more powerful clips. Alternatively, lie on your back with a rock under your shoulders or look for other ways of experimenting with pain.

Next, and importantly, advance to more real-life situations by relinquishing control of the exercises. Get someone else to apply the clips when you are *meditating* and so add the element of the unknown. This will teach you more control over the psychological aspect. Similarly, going outside and sitting near a rotating water sprinkler provides another type of unforeseeable stimulus. Perhaps the ultimate test is *meditating* where flies or mosquitoes are active! Create the opportunities to experience the reality of true pain.

Gain confidence through the exercises, then use your new skill in real life. If you have injections, relax yourself during the procedure and enjoy not having them as hurtful experiences.

I remember well my first trip to the dentist after having resolved my intention of not having an anaesthetic. I felt the techniques should work, but I had yet to test them — to know for sure. Needing a tooth filled, I organised a light workload for the morning of the big day. I made sure that I practised my *meditation* more than usual for days beforehand and practised several times before setting off. Arriving unusually early at the dentist's rooms, I sat and *meditated* some more in his waiting room. My name called, I scampered into the chair to relax myself and get into the *meditation* as quickly as possible. Mumbling that I wanted no anaesthetic the dentist did little to reassure me by replying in a startled voice, 'Are you sure?' Unwaveringly I said I was sure, and the drilling began!

The result amazed me. Not only did I feel no pain, I virtually felt nothing at all. In response to my questions the dentist said that yes, it should have been a painful procedure. The decay was near the tooth's nerve. Definitely I should have felt it. I was elated! For the first time a trip to the dentist had been a positive experience for me. I walked out without half my mouth feeling numb and lop-sided. I had no pain or discomfort whatever, and the tooth was repaired.

I then had a great deal of restorative dental work done, including the fitting of crowns. As I gained confidence I found the 'great *meditation* build-up' was no longer necessary. One morning I managed to cut a finger with an electrical saw. I was lucky I did not cut it off. I sewed up the gaping wound myself without an anaes-thetic. And that same afternoon, I had six fillings in an hour-and-a-half session at the dentist's rooms, again without anaesthetics or any particular preparation. I could feel it all, but there was no pain in it, just a stimulus that for preference I would still rather not have had! And remember, it was not long before this that I was known as having a poor tolerance of pain!

Another happy side effect of these exercises with pain is that they deepen the degree of our *meditation*. Using pain in this way focuses our attention very well and makes sure we are attending to our stated aim. If we do happen to let our mind run free, the pain soon asserts itself and reminds us to get it right. This is a bonus from the exercises that makes them doubly worth practising.

These exercises are ideally done when we feel well. Then we can take our time and there is no urgency to succeed straight away.

But what if pain is already a problem? I am sure that accepting pain as a non-hurtful stimulus is the best way to approach it. The psychological aspect of your pain needs to be understood and treated. However, getting to the point of being able to do that may take some time, training and help. In the meantime, hurtful pain must be alleviated.

Cancer pains can be relieved reliably by external means if you cannot do it yourself. There is no need to feel bad or guilty in seeking such aid. If you are experiencing pain that is above a reasonable threshold for you, it is very appropriate to seek suitable relief. Once the situation is under control you will be able to redevelop your own resources. It is comforting to know that most large centres now boast pain control clinics where the full range of possibilities is explored. One such large clinic in England reported that in one year they admitted four hundred patients with a specific pain problem; only ten could not be relieved satisfactorily.

The range of options used to relieve pain begins with analgesic drugs. They certainly have their place, but can have their problems. Some are addictive, while some affect our normal thinking processes and lessen our quality of life. Practical, non-drug means are preferable. The additional help of counsellors, hypnotherapists, acupuncturists and physiotherapists with mechanical aids such as transcutaneous electrical stimulators may be called for. Even surgeons can contribute by cutting nerves to problem areas.

There are less drastic but more experimental methods which have possibilities. Medical practitioners report consistent pain reduction following large intravenous doses of sodium ascorbate, better known as Vitamin C. Iscador, a German mistletoe extract, has been used by injection, again with considerable results. The controversial laetrile also has been associated with many cases of pain reduction.

At home, I found two great aids, the ever-faithful hot-water bottle applied over the affected area and the generalised effect of caffeine enemas. [More will be said of caffeine enemas in discussing the dietary principles. Also see Appendix C for details of preparation.]

When my pain was really hurting, I found coffee enemas at up to two-hourly intervals gave me good relief. How they work to control pain, I cannot satisfactorily explain. Placebo effect? Well, if that is all they are, it is enough. I do feel sure, however, that there is a physiologically acceptable answer. They worked for me, as they have for many others, and remain worth considering.

Many people have also found that being on a good diet has decreased their perception of pain. Removing any toxic accumulations in the body leads to further reductions. Perhaps this is how the caffeine enemas work as they stimulate the liver's detoxifying processes.

Another very helpful, personal tool, is the radiant light visualisation, described earlier, for once you can picture and feel your body deeply and harmoniously relaxed, pain is greatly lessened.

Other people can also be of great help in the control of your pain. *Touch* works wonders. The comfort produced by a loving hand reaches us on a psychological level and such contact can ease many situations.

Having someone talk through the relaxation we use as a lead-in
to *meditation* can have an even more profound effect. This is a
particularly helpful technique if someone is really distressed. It
works best if the patient's Christian or given name is used while
talking through the exercise. So it could be said: 'Feel your toes,
Ian. Contract the muscles, Ian — and let them go'. The name need
not be used with every phrase, but including it regularly does aid
the process. It should be talked through in a slow, steady unemo-
tional tone and the patient should follow the directions. It should
then finish with an instruction to the patient to imagine that they
are floating comfortably on water. Doing so will reliably produce a
lasting, pain-free calm.

It is worth repeating, again, that relieving muscular tension
through relaxation goes a long way towards relieving pain. The
more relaxed you are, the less pain you will feel.

Of course, you should be working with all the tools discussed
under positive thinking to improve your self-image and level of
well-being. Do not overlook the role of laughing, and indulging
yourself in purely pleasurable activity. Likewise, aim to reach
acceptance of your situation, especially if it does or is likely to
include pain. If you can accept and flow with the pain rather than
resisting and struggling against it, it will cause little inconvenience.

Perhaps the greatest comfort I have gained through my cancer is
learning that true pain does not hurt. Pain is a physical response;
suffering is a conscious reaction which we can choose to do without.

In summary

Causes of pain

A   Physical factors
1   A stimulus warning of physical danger
2   Additional factors
  ● physical tension
  ● toxicity, especially from diet

B   *Psychological causes of pain*
1   Fears
   ● personal
   ● financial
   ● social
2   Self-image: includes
   ● attitudes
   ● expectations
   ● level of well-being
3   Secondary gains
   ● physical
   ● psychological, especially emotional

Treating pain

A   *Personally*
● acceptance
● train with true pain
● diet, enemas
● hot-water bottle
● relaxation
● regular *meditation*
● appreciate psychological loadings and treat with
   positive thinking
   concentration on pleasurable activities
   laughter
   affirmations
   visualisation, especially 'radiant light'

B   *Possible outside help*
● analgesics
● surgery
● counselling
● hypnotherapy
● physiotherapy
● acupuncture
● Vitamin C
● Iscador injection
● touch
● spoken relaxation.

Chapter seven

DIET

The principles – a logical approach

There has to be an appropriate diet that will help cancer patients get well again.

Diet is well established now as a major contributing factor in the development of cancer.

World authority Professor Sir Richard Doll says in his book, *Causes of Cancer*, that the best current estimate is that diet is a major contributing factor in 35 per cent of all cancers.[7] However, medical confirmation of the diet-cancer link has only come in the last few years. Before that time it was vehemently denied in most quarters, as was the thought that diet could help a person to get well. This I cannot understand. A body that is under attack from cancer, whose system may be further stressed by toxic treatments such as chemotherapy and radiation, must have very special demands as it sets about healing itself. More than this, the prospect of diet actually promoting healing is a very real one.

There is an appropriate diet for ulcer patients, kidney patients and heart patients so there *must* be an appropriate diet for cancer patients!

It is a sad fact that in the past most medicos have disagreed with this premise. Now we see a growing level of dietary awareness within society which judges this to have been a short-sighted view and more guidance is being demanded in this area. So there is an emerging number of doctors actively counselling cancer patients on dietary principles. They get results which are plain for all to see, and the interest grows. Yet diet, in the sense in which we are talking, is still frequently, if incredibly, considered to be an 'alternative' area of treatment.

Perhaps this connotation has been helped by the myriads of

specialised diets put forward for just about every condition known to man, and for cancer in particular. At first glance many of these diets appear contradictory and confusing. Some recommend funny things like coffee enemas. What we seek, then, is a rational and reasonable approach to diet. So what general principles can be identified, and how can they be applied on an individual basis?

There is a lot of truth in the old adage, 'You are what you eat'. Your body's performance must be determined by the quality of the fuel it runs on. We use this principle with our motor vehicles so thoroughly. We make sure we use clean petrol of the right grade, we do the same with spark plugs and oil, we get the car regularly cleaned and serviced, and the better we look after it the longer and more efficiently it runs. Just so with the body. Food is our fuel, vitamins our spark plugs. Just as a plodding old pump runs well on diesel, the average car on petrol and a racer on acetone, so individuals and individual situations do best on different fuels. *Recovering from cancer is a very special situation and requires very special food.*

Diet, however, is not the total answer. Just as with any valid medical treatment, the patient's input remains critical. The best diet in the world will not help someone who hates every mouthful. Likewise, we all know happy, symptom-free people who eat pure, unadulterated junk and appear to thrive on it. Happy, eating junk, and thriving? The key word is 'happy', of course. Their level of total health may not be up to its true potential, but there is no doubt that the body does have the remarkable ability to keep going on an enormous range of fuels. People who are well emotionally and mentally have a fair degree of latitude. The body, however, can only compensate so much. It was established by Senator G. McGovern, Chairman of the US Senate Select Committee on Nutrition: Human Needs (1977) that diet contributes significantly to six of the ten major causes of death in modern society: heart disease, diabetes, diverticular disease, obesity, hypertension, and, of course, cancer.

When we aim for optimal health, or even just at prevention of disease, our diet is an area from which we can benefit greatly. With active disease present it becomes a major factor for consideration.

I strongly recommend that any dietary approach should be supervised by a qualified and experienced health professional with the necessary skill and knowledge of nutrition. Ideally, this would be a doctor who fits that description. Some naturopaths may also be suitable. In my experience, patients in a stable condition will find getting their diet organised to be a safe, relatively easy, and certainly rewarding experience. It *is* necessary, however, to be open to change and prepared to learn.

For those in a less stable condition, a word of caution and a repetition: seek suitable, qualified guidance and recognise that you may need to make an intense personal effort to begin with.

For everyone, I suggest that there is the need for a conscious, positive decision regarding diet. Use the decision-making technique:

1 Set a time limit for collecting information on the dietary possibilities.

2 Take what is written here, and add more information from all sources available to you.

3 Assess this body of information.

4 Make a decision and plan a course of action.

5 Commit yourself to a period of time to try your new diet, if you do change anything.

6 At the end of this time, reassess and plan again.

7 Repeat steps 5 and 6, regularly!

There is a great deal that can be done, and remember:

Diet is not the total answer to cancer, but without a good diet there is no answer.

My interest in diets for cancer patients was kindled when my cancer reappeared after the initial surgery and I was told that the normal medical treatments offered little prospect of dealing with it. By a happy chain of events, Grace and I were taken to a lecture on the Gerson diet. We were amazed to find that Dr Max Gerson had an exciting, comprehensive and novel theory on cancer and its dietary treatment. Even better, he had published documented cases of its effectiveness in restoring terminal patients to health in his book. *A Cancer Therapy: with Results of Fifty Cases.*[8]

Gerson was a medical practitioner who had used a dietary

regime to relieve his own otherwise untreatable migraine attacks. He then developed this regime and had good results treating tuberculosis patients with it. He treated his first cancer patient, reluctantly and with little optimism, in 1928. She had a complete remission.

Winston Churchill said, 'Men occasionally stumble over the Truth, but most pick themselves up and hurry off as if nothing had happened'. No doubt Gerson did stumble across this treatment. He, however, spent the next thirty years attempting to validate his results while modifying and improving the diet according to clinical experience.

My feeling from reading Gerson's work is that he had a great faith in nature. He believed that cancer was a multifactorial, degenerative disease. He regarded it as the product of our food and environment being too far removed from nature. He believed that we have exceeded the body's ability to cope with unnatural products. Like me, Gerson saw cancer as a disease of society, a disease of lifestyle. He listed the over-use of artificial fertilisers and chemicals in the soil, the over-refining and adulteration of food with toxic additives, the poor preparation of food and the pollution of our environment generally as being individual factors which combined to adversely affect the body's function as a whole. He postulated that over a period of time these factors weakened the body's resistance to a point where one final trigger-factor produced the localised symptoms.

Approaching as a whole that dynamic, complex system which is the human body is a rapidly growing attitude, but one still novel to many, even today. Yet Gerson was doing this in the 1930s! He was one of the first to suggest that cancer involved the impairment of the body's natural defences, the immune system, in this general-ised way. He was stating, way back then, that cancer involved a problem of immune deficiency. It is only recently that the medical mainstream has begun to explore this avenue and to share this basic concept. Gerson recognised that the theory he worked with, the nutritional basis of his diet and the supplements he used, were subject to medical argument. He was very pragmatic, however. His methods were effective. He preferred to work towards a fully acceptable medical explanation as he continued treating his patients and presenting their favourable results. He claimed a 50 per cent recovery rate, even of terminal cases. There is evidence that he did achieve this remarkable result, made more remarkable by considering that most of his patients had been through the conventional treatments first and gained no success.

Gerson was way ahead of his time. He recognised that once the familiar symptoms of cancer appeared there was a problem which included more than just the localised lumps and bumps. The whole body was diseased. In fact, he stressed that a healthy body could not have cancer.

When thought of, this statement is obvious in the extreme. By definition, a healthy body cannot at the same time be diseased. Often, however, cancer is treated as a localised problem as if it is only the lumps and bumps that are the disease and the rest of the patient's body is fine. It is a new approach to treat the patient as a whole. The exciting extension of thought is that if the rest of the body can be returned to a healthy condition, then it will react to and eliminate any cancer, anywhere in the body.

To test this idea, Gerson did an experiment reminiscent of the kidney transplant case described in Chapter 4. Whereas in that case cancer had been introduced into a healthy body and eliminated, he tried to bring a healthy system to the cancer. Experimentally, he surgically linked the blood supply of a healthy rat to that of a cancerous one. With the healthy blood flowing through its veins, the diseased rat's cancer disappeared.

This, then, was Gerson's aim – to restore the normal function of the body. It fitted my ideas exactly and so I tried it. Having felt its benefits and recognising some of its limitations, I would really like to see a medically supervised trial to evaluate it properly. As far as I know, there has never been one.

It is a very strict and involved regime to follow, and it certainly calls for professional guidance. I tried it with Grace's help, and even with our medically orientated backgrounds we had plenty of problems. I feel that if we had received qualified support at that time, it would have been better for me. As it was, the diet and meditation held my normally agressive type tumours stable for three months, then I deteriorated and had to do many additional things to get free of trouble again.

I certainly recommend *against* anyone trying Gerson's diet on their own. It should really be described as a therapy rather than a diet. As well as the need for supervision and monitoring, there is a need for at least one person to assist with preparation. Grace was involved for about twelve hours each day helping me with it. Obviously the level of commitment needs to be very high on everyone's part. It would not be possible to live a normal life, let alone go to work, while following the diet intensively. It is really a regime best conducted in a live-in clinic situation.

So there are plenty of reservations regarding Gerson's therapy. It is well worth mentioning, however, as his ideas stand on their merits. Also, for those interested in intensive diets, Gerson's is the soundest and best to my knowledge. Most others are adaptations of his.

Finally, by talking of it, a lot of the issues relating to diet can be broached and they certainly warrant consideration. For example, there is a problem with the sense of conflict between the medical profession and those who advocate this type of dietary approach.

On first learning of the diet, it filled me with excitement. Facing a decidedly terminal situation, I was very keen to find an answer. But I sought to maintain an open mind and tried hard to judge the facts critically. The ultimate yardstick is the result that a theory yields.

The woman who first introduced us to Gerson's ideas was a trained nurse. She had inoperable ovarian cancer, multiple metastases, and a six weeks prognosis when she began the therapy. We met her over twelve months later and, while not free of physical problems, she was certainly a joy to meet, an inspiration, and had exceeded all possible medical expectations. She was living proof for us that diet was a significant factor.

Back in 1976, when we tried to share this excitement with my radiotherapist, I was dismissed summarily and told to 'Go home and have a good steak – that will make you feel better!' What disappointed me most was that this same person, while unable to offer any treatment of value, was so ready to discount a diet of which he knew nothing, but the results of which, to me at least, had been substantiated and which I believed just might help. I soon found that those interested in the dietary approach formed almost a counter-culture. Based on their own negative experiences, disillusionment with doctors was rife and cynicism foremost.

Over the years I have been delighted to see this position gradually change. Now there is a growing body of doctors enthusiastic about dietary considerations and prepared to help patients with them on an individual basis. Despite our unique experience and knowledge, we have been reluctant to do this ourselves. Grace and I do not have formal training in the area and we have been keen to avoid difficulties with the authorities. Perhaps this is another limitation we accepted. We feel best talking generalities. Hopefully, we have at least stimulated interest in this vital area. However, we still prefer to leave the specifics to patients to determine in conjunction with those legally qualified to practise. This would seem an appropriate attitude and it works well for our support groups. At the same time in outlining diet as one of the techniques available, we cannot avoid sharing our specific ideas in a book like this.

With Grace helping and also participating, I did follow Gerson's diet rigidly for three months. During this time we both developed a remarkable sensitivity for foods that agreed with us and those which did not. For example, I found eggs disagreed with me. They gave me mild indigestion, a toxic flu-like feeling in the head, and were obviously better avoided.

Over years of modification, based primarily on this sensitivity but backed by all that Grace and I could read and learn on the subject, we have arrived at what we call our maintenance diet. Our diet is born of experience, so we feel it can be justified rationally. It is similar to Pritikin's diet, of which we were unaware until quite recently, and I shall discuss its details in the next chapter.

Meanwhile the specifics of the Gerson approach are best gleaned from his well-written and documented book *A Cancer Therapy – with Results of Fifty Cases.*[9], although, again, I *do not* recommend it. Very few would find it appropriate, taking into account their total situation. It is more beneficial to identify the principles of the dietary approach and to seek a means of applying them in individual cases.

There are four basic principles:

1 The body should be detoxified.

2 Any vitamin and mineral imbalances need to be corrected.

3 The digestion should be restored and flooded with fresh, vital, pure and suitably prepared food.

4 The patient needs to develop and maintain a positive attitude both in a general sense and towards their diet in particular.

1 Detoxification

This is a concept not talked of greatly in medical circles but worth stressing as a starting point. It makes good sense to remove any toxins already in the system and then to avoid introducing any new sources of toxic material. The latter is easier than the former, and can be done by avoiding those things incriminated as having an increased risk of cancer [See list in Chapter 8].

Removing toxins from the body is not such a simple business in theory or practice. It is certainly more open to medical debate. Again, these principles do work, and I suggest they can be validated. It is well known that many toxins, such as those in pesticides, do accumulate in body tissues. When the body has a toxic overload, it can be likened to a system of pipes which are clogged, obstructed and have muddy water flowing through them. The pipes need to be flushed out and clean water introduced into the system. Perhaps this simplistic explanation will appeal more to the gut feeling of patients than to the intellectual, critical analysis of medical staff, but again it seems reasonable.

What is not so reasonable is the emphasis some patients put on detoxifying. Perhaps this is because of feelings of uncleanliness that sometimes accompany disease, but it disappoints me to see some people seeming to delight in detoxifying through cleansing and purging in rather a violent way. Detoxifying is not just cleansing the bowels with gusto! It is a *thorough* spring cleaning for the *whole body* and can be done gently.

Eating a lot of fresh, vital food gets the process in motion. It is accentuated by the use of freshly prepared juices. These Gerson found an ideal source of easily digestible nutrients in a balanced form. Freshly made, they were also full of oxidative enzymes which he believed could help re-oxygenate the cancerous tissue and revitalise the rest of the body. He advocated them on an hourly basis, twelve each day – hence the time commitment for those on his diet. I would recommend the need for moderation, depending upon the individual situation.

Most juices have an acceptable taste, and some are positively pleasant! Orange, apple, grape and carrot are all old favourites. The taste of green juices requires more explanation before they can be relished. Gerson emphasised that the oxidative enzymes in these juices were able to enter into the blood stream and exert a direct effect. Certainly the chlorophyll molecule, the main constituent of green plants, is almost identical to haemoglobin, the main constituent of red blood cells.

Like Gerson, Dr Anne Wigmore has found that using green juices is a great aid to restoring the degenerated metabolism of cancer patients. She used wheatgrass as the main ingredient of her juices. Freshly sprouted wheat is cut off when the shoots are four to five inches high, and juiced. This juice is hard to extract without a specialised juicer, and a good alternative is to chew the shoots, swallow the juice and spit out the fibre – delicately, of course! Gerson, however for his green juices used lettuces, red cabbage leaves, beet tops, swiss chard, green pepper, celery, parsley, etc. and found these to work well.

Gerson also placed great value on raw liver juice. This may sound a trifle revolting, and the taste is certainly nothing to rave over, but again it makes sense. The liver is recognised as the best source of the components that build the blood. Based on its nutrient content, dietitians would certainly rate it as one of the best individual foods. So, why not cook it and eat the whole lot? Why the need to have it as a fresh raw juice? Cooking can affect the vitamins, enzymes, co-factors and other suspected, but as yet unidentified, beneficial substances in liver. Also, the fibre in it is very tough and a cancer patient's digestion is often incapable of dealing with it. It could undergo delayed passage through the bowel, putrefy and then add to the toxicity of the body. So the juice avoids the fibre while saving all the goodness. This juice, like the wheatgrass, is also hard to make, and chewing it in pieces, swallowing the juice and leaving the fibre is a possibility. Chewing raw liver is even less joy than drinking liver juice, so a minimum of cooking – thirty to sixty seconds grilling each side – is a fair compromise. Still spit out that fibre! Sucking a lemon afterwards cleans the palate if the need is there.

Next, the organs of elimination need to be stimulated and assisted in their function. Gerson named the liver as the major organ of detoxification and placed great importance upon restoring and maintaining its efficient activity. He believed the liver juices aided its function and also gave liver extract injections.

His main method for stimulating it, however, was by using caffeine enemas. Caffeine introduced into the rectum by enema is absorbed by the rectal veins into the portal vein, passing from there directly to the liver. There it stimulates bile flow. Bile is a major means of eliminating toxic material from the body.

As coffee is a readily available source of caffeine and also makes a convenient enema, it is coffee enemas that are recommended. I thought it the funniest thing I had ever heard of when it was suggested I should have caffeine enemas. I am sure Spike Milligan's crazy genius could not have produced a more comical idea. But, like everyone else I know who has tried them, I felt an immediate benefit from them and, amidst some hilarity, persisted with them.

While they do hasten elimination, it is to be repeated and emphasised that they are primarily for the liver's benefit. They are also remarkably effective in combating and relieving pain. I found them more useful here than the analgesics I was having when pain was a problem for me. Dr Meares has told me that he believes they have an effect because to hold an enema for ten to fifteen minutes while the caffeine is being absorbed requires quite a degree of relaxation – relaxation in an area you might otherwise not relax so well. I believe this is an added benefit, but they certainly have an immediate physical effect as well. Of all Gerson's treatments, this is the one I kept on with for longest. In the early days, I used to try stopping them and I would become obviously jaundiced in one or two days. A caffeine enema would clear the yellowness from my skin in about fifteen minutes. Again, if the explanation of how they work is inadequate, the pragmatic fact is that many do find them helpful. [See Appendix C for details of preparation and administration.]

Recently Dr Forbes from Bristol has told me that they get just as good results using herbs that stimulate liver function, and they are listed in *A Gentle Way with Cancer*.[10] As these herbs can be taken 'down' rather than 'up', they have a greater aesthetic appeal! Dr Forbes suggests they could be readily included in most situations. He said that unless there was an actual bile obstruction, he knew of no contra-indications. I have no personal experience using these herbs, but Dorothy Hall, Australia's leading herbalist, feels that individual patients require individual treatments. She recommends the seeking of personal advice from a qualified herbalist if you are considering this type of aid. Dandelion root coffee [See page 118] has been recommended for centuries as a liver tonic and we have found it to be a gentle and reliable aid. We recommend its regular use at up to three cups per day. The consideration here is that generally the liver will profit from assistance and it becomes a matter of determining the most appropriate way of providing this.

2   Correct vitamin and mineral imbalances

If you happened to be following Gerson's diet, this question would be easily resolved. The emphasis on fresh foods and juices in his diet provides very high levels of vitamins and minerals in their naturally occurring form. [See Dietary Analysis Appendix A.] He found that adding extra, individual, concentrated vitamin supplements was generally counter-productive. However, he did claim the need for extra amounts of potassium, iodine and niacin (Vitamin B_3). Remember, however, that his diet was an integrated whole. It had been developed through clinical experimentation. By adding and subtracting small parts of the whole and observing the effects, he determined a basic balance that worked. Also, when treating patients, he did modify it to suit individual requirements.

Now, if you are seeking your own balance, the question of supplements is a vexed one indeed. When considering your options, you will find that at one end of the pole are the die-hards who say that none are needed as 'the average diet contains all you need'. At the other end of the spectrum are those who recommend taking vast amounts of every known vitamin, mineral, and just about everything else that can be made into a tablet and swallowed.

What is reasonable? There is good evidence that the 'average' diet is frequently deficient in vital nutrients. A survey examining the vitamin and mineral content of the diets of new patients in a Melbourne medical practice revealed startling results.

The patients whose diets were examined presented for a wide range of everyday problems. They could reasonably be said to represent the average in an affluent society wherein one would expect people to lack little. Yet, even allowing for limitations in the analysis technique, their diets were grossly deficient. And, significantly, the deficiencies showed up in factors directly involved in the normal functioning of the immune system.

The case for supplementation, then, is further increased by the growing body of evidence that large doses of some minerals, and particularly of some vitamins, can be dramatically helpful for some cancer patients.

Vitamin C is in the forefront of this still controversial area. Dual Nobel Prize winner Linus Pauling is probably Vitamin C's most prestigious advocate, and there certainly are many others recommending its use. Looking at the available information on Vitamin C demonstrates the problems surrounding supplements. While some studies say it makes little or no difference, others point to its wide range of beneficial activities. Again, Doctors Pauling and Cameron refer to an increase in the body's natural resistance, in their work *Cancer and Vitamin C*. They cite an improved state of well-being, as measured by improved appetite, increased mental alertness, decreased requirement for pain-controlling drugs, and other clinical criteria.[11]

Most animals make their own Vitamin C. Not so we humans. We rely on our diet for all we get. It has been claimed that an ideal, fresh food diet would provide 8 to 10 grams of Vitamin C daily. Some claim this is a reasonable maintenance level and, ideally, such an amount would be obtained in the diet itself. But, in fact, most people would require supplementation to achieve this level. The official minimum recommended daily allowance is 30 mgms per day. Our maintenance diet contains around 560 mgms per day. Gerson's diet contains 930 mgms.

Another consideration is the level required to bring the body to 'saturation point'. It has been suggested that, at saturation, Vitamin C exerts its maximum effects. It has been suggested that at levels below this its effect may be minimal. To explain: a person in normal health may be at saturation with a total intake of, say, 10 grams. The stress of an impending cold, however, may increase the need for Vitamin C so much that 50 grams may be required to reach saturation. If the person is only getting 10 grams, the cold may develop as normal. Giving 50 grams, however, could prevent it developing at all. Likewise, exposure to 'flu may create a need for 200 grams. Giving 10 or 50 grams would be ineffective, whereas 200 grams would be effective.

It is found that the amount of Vitamin C required to reach saturation varies widely with individuals and individual situations. Doctors working with this approach often use what is called the bowel tolerance test. They find that once the body is saturated, a little extra Vitamin C leads to a mild diarrhoea which stops once the supplementation is reduced a little. This makes the point of bowel tolerance a useful signpost to the individual's maximum requirements. So they recommend that their patients find their own level of bowel tolerance, drop the dose just a little and keep to that, adjusting according to stress levels. Many cancer patients find this requires their adding 18 to 20 grams of Vitamin C to their diet daily. Some take 30 grams or more by mouth each day. Such high levels of Vitamin C are said to leach magnesium, zinc and Vitamin B6 from the body, and so supplements of these are then required.

Often even higher doses of Vitamin C are given intravenously with some good effects. A common, almost uniform result, is the lessening of pain. Some tumours also do regress. I have treated confirmed cases of lymphosarcoma in cats with intravenous doses of 1 gram per kilogram of body weight on five successive days. Four out of four treated cases have gone into total remission. Dogs I have treated in the same manner have not responded so well.

The special case of Vitamin C amply demonstrates the complex and really rather confusing issues involved with supplements.

I hope it is obvious that I am only discussing the options, and avoiding making specific recommendations. Supplements pose many complex questions. Their role is not one I find easy to resolve.

My own experience with them runs the full gamut. I did take all the supplements Gerson recommended when I was trying his regime. His was an integrated approach. I then dropped various factors off as I began to feel them unnecessary, relaxing towards our Maintenance Diet. At another time I tried mega-vitamin therapy – taking huge numbers of vitamin tablets. Apart from learning the art of swallowing thirty pills in one go, I felt it did little for me. Yet, at specific times, I have felt the need for specific supplements and benefited from them. Now I take none except the occasional multi-vitamin. If my throat feels inflamed, or I get stressed as with air travel, I take large doses of Vitamin C and a supplement that provides the main vitamins and minerals involved with the immune system. This keeps me free of problems and I rarely need to take them for more than a day or two.

My overriding attitude is that natural sources are best. Ideally our diet should provide the range of nutrients we require for optimal health and healing. I doubt that this often occurs. The range of supplements that can or should be considered as being useful is wide indeed. Doctors using them with cancer patients draw on Vitamins A, B, C and E, potassium, iodine, zinc, selenium and so on. So supplements are a difficult question, the one I find the hardest to be clear about and I make no definite recommendations. However, I do feel confident of a diet I have developed to use in cases of small animals with cancer [See Appendix D]. I find that this diet, in conjunction with its supplements dramatically and consistently improves the animal's quality of life. Owners regularly report that their old dogs are behaving like puppies again, full of life, vigour and happiness. Only occasionally have we found that the diet stops the cancer or puts that patient into remission. However, the animals certainly enjoy themselves and the owners are happy that they can, in fact, do something constructive. We also find that when the end does come it is not a long drawn-out affair. There is usually good quality of life until a point is reached when a rapid decline sets in. This again makes the situation easier to cope with.

So which supplements, if any, should be used by human cancer patients, and at what levels, is a matter for determination by qualified personnel who can evaluate individual circumstances.

A difficult task, as this is an emerging area, and I suggest there are as yet no easy answers. As more doctors work in this field and evaluate their results, the facts will become more obvious and so recommendations can be more concrete. [This is dealt with in more detail in Chapter 8.]

3 Restore the digestion

Here again the idea of supplementing the digestive functions is medically questionable. I find this easier to put forward as there is little doubt that most cancer patients initially do have an impaired digestion. Gerson recommended supplementing stomach acid and pancreatic enzymes. There have been several claims that pancreatic enzymes can actually attack cancer cells and digest them. I

find the evidence for this to be sketchy. It is hard to imagine such
supplements doing harm, however, and there is a body of circum-
stantial evidence which suggests that they might do good. I took
them while on Gerson's therapy but they were one of the first
things I discontinued.

4 *Restore and maintain a positive attitude*

This whole area of diet is full of excitement, controversy and the
definite prospect of being helpful. It is essential to be clear in your
own mind as to the relevance it has for you. You should feel good
about your choices. It is very necessary to think about the whole
area and to come to definite conclusions. In the final analysis food
should be a happy thing. You should be able to sit down before it,
give thanks for what you have to eat, know that it is appropriate
for your situation, and eat it with a smile on your lips and a song in
your heart!

Chapter eight

DIET

The practice – good food and how to prepare it

As we begin converting the principles of diet into practice, there is no way we can avoid the necessity to talk specifics. I stress again the need for individualised professional guidance in this matter. While it would be most evasive of me to avoid putting forward our general ideas, you must please realise that these are *not* blanket recommendations. I can give a range of options as we see them. Let *this* range of options merely contribute to the spectrum of information on which you can base your *own* decisions. I cannot make those decisions for you.

Do be warned by the example of Ernie. Ernie made his own investigations, became enthused about diet and followed one most conscientiously. The problem was, what he chose was quite inappropriate for him. Ernie had had his stomach removed. On the diet he chose his special requirements were not even nearly met and, as a consequence, he had to spend time in hospital to recover from his enthusiasm. There is the need for caution, so please do seek professional help in order that you can be monitored and guided.

In the last chapter we examined some of the dietary theories advanced and identified several principles. That was the easy part! The next challenge is to seek a means of transposing these principles into practice. There would seem to be four alternatives:

1 Make no change
2 Adopt the Maintenance Diet
3 Follow the Individual Restoration Programme
4 Commit yourself to a specific intense diet such as Gerson's and seek professional help with it – preferably in a suitable clinic.

1   *Make no change*

If you are happy with your diet as it is and feel it cannot be improved, that is fine. Skip the rest of this chapter and go on with the other things available to help you back to health.

I am convinced that dietary considerations are one of the the basic tools for getting well. Also, most of the dietary factors associated with a risk of increasing the incidence of cancer are prominent in our Western diet. These factors are a high content in the diet of fat, protein, salt, sugar, refined foods and foods with a low fibre content, as well as too many calories, smoking nicotine and drinking excessive alcohol. It is likely, then, that most people need to consider making changes. A suitable approach would be to take on one of the following possibilities:

2   *The Maintenance Diet*

This is a relatively easy step. It requires eliminating from the diet those things associated with a health risk and concentrating on what is left. In general terms, then, the ideal diet is low in fat and protein, has no salt, sugar, refined foods or nicotine, but a little alcohol is acceptable. It concentrates on the basic food groups of fruit, vegetables and grains. For many people, then, this type of diet does involve a great change in eating habits, but it still fits readily into most daily routines. It would be excellent for those who are in a stable condition to begin with or for anyone interested in both preventing disease and in maximising their health. I feel confident in putting it forward as a basic, sensible and sound diet.

So first we list the things to avoid. Let it be said that the level of risk associated with some of these factors is very much open to debate. Fluoride is probably the best example, where emotional issues seem to govern people's decisions as much as the arguable facts. While there is good evidence that it helps prevent dental caries, the evidence that it is carcinogenic is slim indeed.

My attitude is that if there is doubt about any factor, and it is practical to do so, then it is wise to leave it out of your routine. There is no doubt that dietary factors are important, but scientifically proving which ones, and to what degree, remains a difficulty. Research in this area is picking up momentum now, and hopefully the ensuing years will give a more definitive list. For the present, then, if there is doubt about a factor, I would rather leave it alone and let someone else find out if it is a problem.

An added reason to avoid suspected factors is that they often interact with each other to produce greatly increased risk factors. This is amply demonstrated by the work done on smoking tobacco. Someone who smokes 30 grams of tobacco or more a day has about eight times the risk of oesophageal cancer compared to someone who does not smoke. Drinking 40 to 80 grams of alcohol per day results in seven times the risk of oesophageal cancer compared with someone who does not. Now, if a person does both, what is their risk? Eight plus seven, or fifteen times greater? Unequivocably no! The evidence is clearcut. The two risks don't simply add together – the effect is more like multiplication. The combined risk of smoking and drinking together, at that level, is put at thirty-six times that of doing neither.

Similarly, asbestos workers who smoke get ten times the incidence of asbestosis compared with those who do not. Cigarette smokers in the cities have twice the lung cancer of their country counterparts. What extra factors are involved here? Pollution? Stress?

It seems highly likely that this compounding effect of carcinogens operates in other areas. I feel it will be shown to be a major cause in producing cancer, and the reason why we should attend to our diet and environment closely, seeking to make it as pure as practicable.

There are so many things in common usage that are known to have a risk factor or are suspected of having one. We have listed all we currently know about, with suggestions on what steps can be taken to avoid them altogether or substitute for them.

Foods and Other Factors to Avoid

Avoid	Comments	What to do
High FAT intake	Strong link between high intake and breast cancer (where milk fat shows a particularly high link) and endometrial cancer. Always bad, but more so if fats are overheated and/or rancid. Rancidity occurs in any fat or oil that is exposed to prolonged heat/air/light, e.g.	1 tablespoon cold pressed vegetable oil (we use olive) per day is maximum to add to diet. Avoid other sources of high fat, e.g. animal fat. (See special section on dairy products in this Chapter and individual sources of fats/oils in vegetable listings.)
	1 Oils used for repeated frying.	Avoid deep frying with the same oil. Preferably sauté with water instead of frying and use oils that are most stable if you do use them, e.g. butter (preferably) or olive oil.
	2 Oils overheated in cooking.	Avoid cooking with oils. Olive is the most stable. Add them after cooking.
	3 De-hulled nuts and seeds.	Ideally buy nuts in shells. Don't use de-hulled sunflower seeds etc. that have had long storage times. (See Nuts in this Chapter.)
	4 Wheatgerm oil begins rancidifying one week after processing.	Don't use it.
	5 Flour begins rancidifying three days after milling.	Use your own home flour mill or obtain flour freshly ground at health food store, co-op., etc.
	6 Vegetable oils stored in clear containers.	Buy them in amber glass or tin containers.

Avoid	Comments	What to do
High SALT intake	No extra is needed in cooking or at table. (Possible exception being people who work hard in hot weather and sweat profusely.)	Leave it out and watch your taste buds redevelop. Or, substitute by using Vitamin C (sodium ascorbate) in equivalent amounts.
High SUGAR intake	Sugars including other refined carbohydrates are the empty calories and should be avoided.	About 1 teaspoonful of natural honey or pure maple syrup is daily maximum.
High PROTEIN* intake	Meat is better avoided as there is a link with colo-rectal cancer particularly. Especially incriminated are red meat, sausage meat, and barbecued meat.	There are many low protein sources in the diet which add to the overall total, e.g. grains. Add to this a maximum of 1.5 kilograms total per week taken from the following high protein sources, listed in descending order of preference (e.g. vegetable protein sources are preferable, fatty meats are highly undesirable): 1. Vegetable proteins: soy beans, tofu or bean curd, lentils, chick peas, any of the beans or peas (known collectively as legumes or pulses); 2. Fish (preferably small deep sea ones). Eggs (3 per week if agreeable; duck eggs may be suitable if hen eggs are not), dairy products, yoghurt especially, low fat cow's milk if suitable, soft cheeses. Goat's milk (which we use) may be suitable if cow's milk is not; 3. Meat, descending order again: lean white meat, rabbit, veal, free range chicken, lean red meat, fatty meats.

Avoid	Comments	What to do
High ALCOHOL intake	Probably better avoided but a small amount can help stimulate Prostaglandin E1 which aids immune function.	½ 'pint' of beer, or 2 glasses of wine, or 2 tots of spirits, is maximum.
Smoking TOBACCO	This is a self-destructive habit – find a better one! 30 per cent of all cancers are directly attributable to smoking. 140,000 people died in America in 1981 as a result of smoking.	Stop: Find a more appropriate way of gaining pleasure and dealing with stress.
Low FIBRE intake	Fibre hastens elimination and its bulk protects the bowel from many problems.	Always use wholemeal grains. Do not peel vegetables, merely wash and scrub with brush.
Bad COOKING techniques	Smoked food, charcoal broiling, barbecuing, can all cause pyrolysis and lead to production of dangerous polycyclic hydrocarbons.	Use steaming, dry baking, Chinese style wok cooking, or cook over a low heat with minimal water which should not be discarded. Do not eat food which has been burnt black.
AFLATOXINS	A fungus that can contaminate peanuts especially, and other carbohydrates – mostly in tropical areas and is linked with liver cancer. Effect probably is increased by Hepatitis B virus.	Restrict use of peanuts unless aflatoxin levels are known. Peanuts are also high in oil and are probably best avoided or kept for special occasions only. Avoid any part of food with signs of fungus or mould on it anywhere. (Such growth may not be aflatoxious, but can be dangerous.)
CAFFEINE	As in coffee, tea, chocolate. A controversial area but, in balance, we prefer to avoid them.	Use herb teas, fruit juices, etc. It is also wise to avoid other artificial soda drinks.

Avoid	Comments	What to do
ARTIFICIAL SWEETENERS	e.g. saccharine. Again, the evidence is unclear, but doubts continue.	Go without, or use a little honey.
CHEMICAL ADDITIVES to food	Some artificial colourings are still used in Australia despite being removed from U.S. markets because of possible associated risks. Flavourings such as monosodium glutamate are suspect, as are some preservatives, particularly the nitrites. There are too many doubts about chemical additives and it is practical to avoid them.	**Read labels.** Aim to eat fresh, whole unprocessed food. If not always practicable, it is preferable to avoid chemical additives **but** make sure the food has been properly stored or preserved. There is good evidence that adequate use of preservatives and refrigeration actually decreases the incidence of stomach cancer. Use suitable herbs and seasonings but avoid regular use of hot spices, chili, commercial mustards and sauces.
PESTICIDE RESIDUES on food	A huge range of chemicals is used and it is not possible that the effects of all of them are fully understood.	Seek out organically grown food and encourage its supply. The less chemical unknowns in your diet, the better.
FLUORIDE in water	Is helpful for children's teeth but questionable for cancer patients.	Preferably use spring or rain water. Consider a purifier for your mains water.
CHLORINATION of water	Possibly linked with cancer of bladder and large intestine.	As above.
VITAMIN, MINERAL and ENZYME DEFICIENCIES		Vitamins A, C and E and selenium appear to have cancer-protective factors and should be high in the diet. They are found naturally in whole grains and in yellow and green leafy vegetables. A healthy person on this diet should not need supplements.

Avoid	Comments	What to do
Excess ALUMINIUM intake	There is no clearcut evidence, but many questions and doubts persist concerning aluminium cookware and deodorants which may contain up to 20 per cent aluminium.	Use stainless steel, glass, enamel, cast iron, earthenware or tin cookware. **Read labels.**
OVER-NUTRITION	The overweight get more cancer than lean people.	Eat only when necessary! Better to under-eat than over-eat. Most people on this type of diet tend to a lean optimal weight.
CHEMICAL CARCINOGENS	e.g. Oestrogen (DES), polycyclic hydrocarbons (coal tar, dyes, etc.), most hair dyes, phenacetin, vinyl chloride (used to make PVC), certain forms of arsenic, cadmium, chromium, nickel, dichlorvos (as in some pet collars and pest strips).	There is inadequate knowledge concerning the safety of many chemicals in current use. Without being paranoid, it is wise to be as careful as practicable. A good reference is *Cancer Causing Agents* by R. Winter. (See Further Reading list.)
IONISING RADIATION	1 Excessive exposure to sunlight (ultraviolet rays are the problem and cause skin cancer).	Avoid sunburn. Use sun-screen lotions. Sunbathe before 11 a.m. and after 3 p.m. Fair-haired, pale-skinned people in the tropics require extra caution to avoid excess sun contact.
	2 Excessive X-rays. Any X-ray is associated with a risk – the more X-rays, the more risk.	While modern X-rays have low exposure, their benefits need to be weighed against the risk. Pregnant women and young children should be extremely careful.

Avoid	Comments	What to do
	3 Fluorescent lighting. Recent evidence suggests that prolonged exposure may increase the risk of melanoma.	Where possible, use natural forms of lighting, e.g. sunlight, globes, or full spectrum fluorescent lights.
	4 Leakage from microwave ovens.	Most modern microwave ovens do not have this problem but we prefer not to use them because we do not like the idea of radiating our food.
	5 Exposure to radio-active material.	Press for an end to nuclear testing!
	6 Television and computer screens.	It is wise to avoid watching too much television, and do not sit close to or directly in front of the set.
POLLUTION	Particularly the end-products from the combustion of fossil fuels are suspect.	Be aware of caring for your environment.
SEXUAL EXCESSES	Too much or too little is a problem! Late age at first child's birth (parity), zero or low parity, and promiscuity are all associated with increased risk.	Moderation in all things.
LOW LEVEL of EXERCISE and POOR GENERAL HEALTH	Chronic infections and a generally low level of resistance or immunity frequently precede cancer.	Exercise appropriately (See Chapter 5) and take adequate preventive measures. There is more to health than just being symptom-free. Work towards optimal health.
STRESS	An inability to cope with stress appropriately is a common factor in most cancer patients' lives. (See Chapter 9)	Avoid stress where possible as you learn to cope with it. *Meditation* and positive thinking work wonders.

107

Some individual items that are included in the maintenance diet are not suitable for someone in an unstable condition. For example, vegetables that need to be cooked, or fruits that have a high fat content, may be eaten only occasionally in an acute condition but may be quite suitable for regular use in the maintenance diet.

For patients in an acute condition, we suggest concentrating on raw food, particularly in summer, until the situation stabilises. Hence the different recommendations to the maintenance diet. We feel confident that the maintenance diet is a good baseline for most people, certainly for those who are basically healthy and want to get the best value from their food. Also, most patients will find this a good starting point, one that will provide most of the benefits that nutrition has to offer.

The lists that follow show how and when we would use each food, including their suitability for juicing, raw food, steaming or baking. Any worthwhile comments have been added.

These lists are based on our experience and the knowledge we have gleaned from reading as widely as we can. However, we offer them as an introductory guide only. Each should pursue their own research, using these lists as a starting point.

List of Vegetable uses

Vegetable	Acute	Maintenance	Preparation*	Comments
*J = juice R = raw S = steam B = bake Sa = sauté in water, wok				
Artichokes Globe	Yes	Yes	S	
Jerusalem	Yes	Yes	S B	Good for diabetics. Low allergenic food.
Asparagus	Yes	Yes	S Sa	Highly recommended.
Beetroot	Yes	Yes	J R S B	Good blood builder. Combines well with other juices.
Beetroot tops	Yes	Yes	J R S	Do have a little oxalic acid, but a good source of potassium.
Broccoli	Occasional	Yes	R S Sa	All Brassicas are associated with cancer protecting factors.
Brussels sprouts	Occasional	Yes	S Sa	Brassica
Cabbage	Yes	Yes	R S Sa	Brassica. Small amount of cabbage juice is good for ulcers and upset stomachs. Is acid-forming. Can be gas-producing, especially for older people – not so bad steamed.
Capsicum	Yes	Yes	J R S Sa B	Red has more Vitamin C than green. Juice good for sore throat.
Carrot	Yes	Yes	J R S B Sa	Excellent juice. Highly recommended. Source of Vitamin A. Combines well with other juices.
Cauliflower	Occasional	Yes	R S Sa	Brassica. Caution with gas if raw. Good source of calcium.
Celery	Yes	Yes	J R S Sa	Good source of potassium, especially the tops. Excellent tonic for urinary system.
Chicory	Yes	Yes	R S	Steam in other greens.

109

Vegetable	Acute	Maintenance	Preparation*	Comments
Chili	No	No		Too stimulating.
Choko	Occasional	Yes	S B Sa	
Cucumber	No	Occasional	J R	Juice aids treatment of kidney and gall stones. Acid-forming.
Eggplant	No	Occasional	S B Sa	Can aggravate arthritic conditions. Member of Solanum family – caution.
Garlic	Occasional	Occasional	R S Sa	Good condiment, flavouring, dressing. One clove of garlic in carrot juice works well. Worm treatment. Blood cleanser. Can be pickled. Sauté leads to less aromatic acids. Chelating agent for heavy metals. Recommended for chemotherapy patients. Regulates blood pressure. Has anti-cancer properties.
Ginger	Yes	Yes	J R	Use sparingly, but excellent additive to vegetables, particularly for vegetarians. Good to stimulate stomach acid and spleen function. Can add to carrot juice. Use for flavouring.
Horseradish	Yes	Yes	R	Aids lung conditions, emphysema. Condiment.
Kohl rabi	Occasional	Yes	B	
Leek	Occasional	Yes	S Sa B	
Mushroom	No	Occasional	R Sa	(Cook on low heat with little water.)
Okra	Occasional	Yes	S Sa	
Onion	Occasional	Occasional	R S Sa B	High in aromatic acids. Good for helping with weight reduction. Better cooked than raw.

Vegetable	Acute	Maintenance	Preparation*	Comments
Parsnip	Occasional	Yes	S B	High calcium source.
Potatoes: Common	Yes	Yes	S B	Skins good for potassium. Solanum. Baked especially recommended.
Potatoes: Sweet	Occasional	Yes	S B	
Pumpkin	Yes	Yes	R S B	Easily digested. Vitamin A, zinc, and aids digestion (natural source of pancreatic type enzymes).
Pumpkin seeds	Yes	Yes	R S B	Excellent for zinc.
Radish	Yes	Yes	R	Stimulant – use moderately.
Silver beet	Yes	Yes	J R S	High oxalic acid content – use 2-3 times per week at maximum.
Spinach	Yes	Yes	J R S	High oxalic acid content – use 2-3 times per week at maximum.
Squash	Occasional	Yes	R S B	
Swede	Occasional	Yes	S B	
Sweet corn	Yes	Yes	R S B	Can be baked in husk (250°C).
Tomato	Yes	Yes	J R S B Sa	Solanum. Excellent source of Vitamin C, 1 gram per large naturally ripened tomato. (Acid-free variety available – Tom Thumb, Roma).
Turnip	Occasional	Yes	S B	
Water cress	Yes	Yes	J R	Good for arthritis.
Zucchini	Yes	Yes	R S B Sa	

List of fruit uses

Fruit	Acute	Maintenance	Preparation*	Comments
Apple	Yes	Yes	J R B Sa	Cook in juice or water.
Apricot	Yes	Yes	J R Sa	Good sun-dried (soak before eating). Kernels can be source of B_{17}, eaten with fruit. Start with 5, add 1 each day up to 15 or, if headache occurs, decrease.
Avocado	No	Occasional	R B	High fat content. Taste terrific!
Banana	Yes	Yes	R B	Potassium. Gentle on upset stomach. Common allergen. Eat when ripe.
Berries including strawberries	No	Occasional	J R Jam	Make into jam with honey. Blood builders. Acidity can be a problem.
Cherry	Yes	Yes	J R Sa	Good source of iron.
Citrus fruits	Yes	Yes	J R	Oranges, grapefruit, limes, mandarins, lemons. Care with acidity. Dilute juices at least 50:50. Good to start day with.
Fig	Occasional	Occasional	R S	High sugar. Excellent laxative.
Grapes	Yes	Yes	J R	Very good blood cleanser. Excellent tonic. See grape diet. Red grapes build blood, white cleanse intestines.
Mango	Yes	Yes	J R	Very palatable!
Melons	Yes	Yes	J R	Cantaloup, water melon, honey dew. Good kidney tonics. Eat on own – not with other fruits, foods. (See Food Combinations later in this Chapter.)

112

Fruit	Acute	Maintenance	Preparation*	Comments
Nectarine	Yes	Yes	J R S	
Papaya	Yes	Yes	J R	Excellent source of papain, digestive enzyme.
Passionfruit	Yes	Yes	R S	
Peach	Yes	Yes	J R S	
Pear	Yes	Yes	J R S	
Persimmon	Yes	Yes	R	Must be ripe.
Pineapple	No	Occasional	J R	Have bromelain, an enzyme reputed by some to take the outer layer off tumours. But, care with acidity.
Plum	Yes	Yes	J R S	
Prune	Yes	Yes	J R S	Laxative. Improves blood iron.
Rhubarb	No	Very occasional	S	High oxalic acid content.

113

Dairy products

Cow's milk is high in fat content and is a very common source of food allergy. It frequently produces sinusitis, persistent sore throats and ear abscesses in young children. Grace suffered sinusitis and cystitis for many years before identifying her severe cow's milk allergy. For some, but not all, goat's milk is a viable alternative.

For maintenance, we recommend cutting dairy products out of the diet for a period (from two weeks to two months. You need to be very thorough as dairy products are added to a wide range of prepared foods) and then reintroducing them. If there is any adverse reaction, try goat's milk or soy products.

For acute patients, our experience is that the majority feel better without dairy products, and so that is the basic recommendation. They can be introduced on a trial basis once maintenance is established.

Cheese; the cottage types are best in all situations, leaving the hard cheeses for special occasions. Camembert's taste adds to its claim to occasional use!

Skim milk or full cream? Pritikin says that cow's milk when left to stand, settles and the cream should then be discarded in the same way we peel an orange. My basic preference is still for whole foods and at home we use goat's milk, which does not aggravate Grace's allergy and is naturally homogenised. However, if we were to use cow's milk products, I would prefer the skimmed or low fat types.

Yoghurt. An excellent addition to the diet in small amounts. It is easily digested and has the same beneficial bacteria as the bowel should normally contain. For people on most types of chemotherapy or undergoing radiation of the abdomen, the effect of reseeding the normal bowel flora with the regular use of yoghurt is very beneficial in stabilising bowel action. We recommend up to two tablespoonfuls per day be used.

In summary: At home we do use goat's milk yoghurt daily, goat's milk cottage cheese regularly, and just small amounts of fresh goat's milk in hot drinks occasionally. Grace has to avoid all cow's milk products and the only ones I have would be some cheese, very occasionally and usually in cooking when we are out. I love Camembert and eat it very occasionally.

Eggs

We consistently find that cancer patients who become sensitive to what agrees with them find that eggs do not. This is probably largely an allergy problem, but also they seem to place heavy demands on the liver for digestion. Many patients report feeling "liverish" after eating eggs. I feel quite "off" after eating hen eggs but I can eat two or three duck eggs a week. Apparently they have different enzymes to the hen eggs and so can be an alternative.

Again we recommend leaving eggs out for two to eight weeks, and reintroducing them to see the effect. In the acute phase we feel they are better avoided. In maintenance, two to four per week is reasonable. The cholesterol issue is not a problem if the eggs are part of the overall maintenance diet.

Seek to use free-range eggs.

Meat

In the acute phase most patients feel better without it, relying on vegetable proteins. We see this most clearly when so many patients do go without it for one to two months as recommended and then re-introduce it. Many do not feel so good and so prefer to stay off it.

For many years we have been conditioned to believe that a high protein, high meat diet was good. Now it is increasingly obvious that the reverse is true. It seems that a high meat, low fibre diet is particularly detrimental. One view of this is that man, being an omnivore, is just not designed for it. A carnivore, being designed to eat meat, has a short digestive tract and a low transit time, that is, a meal eaten this morning will be passed out six to eight hours later. A herbivore, designed to eat herbage and vegetables, has a long digestive tract and a long transit time – two to even four days passing before the grass does also! Man, being an omnivore is trying to get the best of both worlds! We have an intermediate length digestive tract which aims to retain vegetables long enough for digestion, but which does not retain meat so long that it putrefies.

A *low* fibre diet leads to an increased transit time and less protection of the bowel through the buffer action of the fibre's bulk. If you want to check your transit time, eat a little raw millet and see how long it takes to reappear in the toilet. It should be under twenty-four hours – preferably around eighteen hours.

A slow transit time, coupled with a high meat diet, gives the meat wastes the opportunity to putrefy. Direct irritation is then thought to account for the increase in lower bowel disease associated with the low fibre, high meat diet.

For this reason we recommend vegetable proteins as being more suitable for optimum health than animal proteins. Certainly in the acute phase of cancer, most patients in our experience, feel better without it. We generally recommend leaving it off the menu for one to two months and then reintroducing it. When doing so, many patients have felt the worse for it and so have chosen to not eat meat.

If you do choose to use it, remember that the meat should be the condiment to the rest of the meal. The maximum is one half to three-quarters of a kilogram per week. (Remember that this total must include other sources of high protein also.)

Sources: lean, white meat is best; veal, rabbit (being free range rabbit should be excellent!) and chicken (if free-range). There has to be a better way to raise food than in a battery. If it came to a choice of eating or not eating a battery hen, I would rather eat its pellets and save the bird the trouble. If eating red meat, choose lean meat, avoiding fat wherever possible. The fatty meats like hamburger and pork should be at the end of the list.

Cooking: ways that avoid the fat are best, e.g. rotisserie or grilling.

Fish

Minimal in acute phase, suitable for maintenance. We eat fish once a week or fortnight. We have not had it at home for years, but eat it when dining out.

It is preferable to eat small, deep-sea fish, if practical, as these accumulate less pollutants. Shell fish, which do tend to accumulate pollutants, should be kept for very special occasions.

Juices

These are an excellent source of readily absorbed nutrients in a balanced form. Highly recommended in the acute phase, particularly. Ideally six to seven 200 ml (7-oz) juices can be taken daily: start the morning with citrus (orange or half lemon/half water) then have apple, grape, carrot, beetroot, and one or two green juices. Apple and grape can be bought if pure organically grown juices are available, while the others are best made freshly. The carrot and beetroot can be combined. The green juices can be made from a combination of celery, green pepper, lettuce, a *little* cabbage, a little silver beet or spinach, and a little parsley. Wheatgrass is another option, and is discussed in Chapter 7. If you use wheatgrass, begin with 60 ml (2 oz) per day (you may like to dilute it with water) and build to five to seven ozs daily over 7 to 10 days.

Juice machines. The normal commercial juicer uses a centrifugal action which shreds the food, then spins it at high speed. This is a fine way to separate the pulp from the juice, and the juice is packed with nutrients, vitamins and minerals. It is claimed, however, that the centrifugal action of these machines creates a static electricity which destroys the oxidative enzymes in the juice. Gerson asserted this and claimed he saw better results when using a machine that had no static in it. He recommended a machine that separately grinds and then presses the juices out by hydraulic action. Fine in theory but expensive in practice. The Norwaulk machine he preferred now costs well in excess of $1,000. The Champion juicer seems like a reasonable alternative, costing under $500 and being like a mechanised meat-mincer in action. These machines do also extract more juice from the same amount of ingredients than the standard machines. So, if you are serious about juices, I think they are worth considering.

Herbs to consider – an introduction to our favourites.

Most herbs have definite medicinal properties and should be used wisely.

Blood purifiers: This group of herbs are all renowned as blood cleansers or purifiers. They can be used regularly by cancer patients for making teas:
Alfalfa, Red Clover, Chaparral, Nettle, Marshmallow, Comfrey.
Combinations can be used, and a particularly good one is *alfalfa, red clover, marshmallow and comfrey.*

Comfrey is also known as 'knit-bone', as it helps broken bones to heal. It has many other good properties, but used fresh and to excess it causes liver problems. Dried for tea it does not have this difficulty.

Any of the *mints* make a good refreshing drink and can be used cold in summer. They have a tannin content, so do not overdo them. *Peppermint* is particularly useful to aid digestion. soothe the bowel and decrease flatulence.

Camomile, a mild sedative, aids sleep, soothes upset stomach and bowel, and decreases flatulence.

Colt's foot is excellent for chest complaints, particularly if mucus needs to be cleared – it is a good expectorant. Prepare by adding two tablespoonfuls of leaves to one pint of boiling water, stand for about ten minutes, strain, add one teaspoonful of honey and the juice of a quarter of a lemon. Drop the squeezed lemon into the drink also.

Dandelion root coffee is an excellent liver tonic. A cup each day is well worth considering. Use the root for preference. Boil or percolate as for normal coffee, and strain. Add honey or milk if preferred and suitable.

Seasonings

Garlic has been shown to be a natural antibiotic and anti-fungal agent, to decrease blood pressure, to have anti-cancer properties, and is a chelating agent. Like garlic, ginger also makes an excellent seasoning while having special properties. It stimulates stomach acid production, so aiding digestion. Ginger is particularly useful for people changing from a heavy meat based diet to a more vegetarian way of eating.

Other acceptable seasonings are allspice, anise, bay leaves, celery seeds, coriander, dill, fennel, mace, marjoram, rosemary, sage, saffron, tarragon, thyme, and summery savoury.

Ferments

These are often recommended, but apart from yoghurt they are not things we used or use. Sauerkraut is high in lactic acid and is fine if you want to use it. Rejuvelac is a ferment of wheat which is high in active enzymes and can be taken regularly. (See Appendix B for details of preparation.)

Legumes or Pulses

This includes the many different peas and beans

Raw: Eat raw or cook as any other vegetable. Examples: french beans, runner beans, peas, snow peas.

Dried: Examples: soya, kidney, lima and mung beans, chick peas, lentils. These are the seeds of the plant; they are easy to store, a good source of carbohydrate and protein – especially when combined with equal amounts of rice, wheat, etc. They require special cooking as uncooked they contain alkaloids and glycosides which are detrimental to digestion, so never eat them raw. Sprouting them first is ideal, but this takes 2 to 4 days. They do need eight to sixteen hours soaking in water and then simmering until cooked – usually for two hours. (With lentils you must throw out the soaking water and replace it before boiling.) Another cooking method is to pour boiling water over the beans, allow to soak two hours, then cook as above.

Sprouts

Should be an integral part of the diet. We use them daily and prepare them ourselves. Add half a centimetre of alfalfa seeds to the bottom of a 1 kg. jar. Cover well with water and leave soaking for eight hours. Cover the jar with flywire, holding it on with a rubber band. Invert the jar, pouring off the water. Rinse and drain twice. Store upside down. We use a rack I built for the purpose which sits on our kitchen bench, away from direct sunlight. Rinse thoroughly with water twice, both morning and evening (three times in hot weather). In 4-5 days the seeds will have sprouted and be nearly an inch long with little green heads. We always have four jars at various stages of development as our family devours the contents of one each day. They are an ideal source of fresh, vital food, especially in winter. They are meant to be one of the highest sources of vegetable protein and are packed with vitamins and minerals. Highly recommended.

Supplements of vitamins and minerals

The possibilities:

1   Rely on natural sources, e.g., good food and juices. This is our preference.

2   Follow specific recommendations from qualified personnel. These usually fall into two approximate groups:
(a) Supplement the immune system with a single tablet intended for this purpose, e.g., *Bioglan Formula 4.* This contains: Vitamin A 3000 I.U., Vitamin C 250 mgm, Vitamin E 80 I.U., Vitamin B$_6$ 50 mgm, Vitamin B$_5$ 50 mgm, Vitamin B$_2$ 10 mgm, Folic Acid 50 mgm, Magnesium orotate 50 mgm, Zinc chelate 100 mgm, Copper chelate 7.5 mgm, Iron chelate 5 mgm, and Manganese 5 mgm in a low allergy base. They are recommended at one tablet three times daily for adults.

(b) More intensive supplementation. I spoke with a medical practitioner who treats many cancer patients and has the attitude that nutrition and supplements can help to maximise the patient's potentials. His opinion is that the supplements are worthwhile and do produce direct benefit. This he believes is particularly noticeable for patients under the added stress of chemotherapy and radiation where not only are there greater demands placed on the body's resources but its ability to absorb nutrients is often impaired. He provided the following example of his recommendations and explains that he feels these things are interdependent and make for a total approach, that is it is all or nothing with these supplements.

Vitamin A: 8 drops twice daily of Micelle A (Bioglan). This is equivalent to 18-20,000 I.U. An overdose of Vitamin A produces headache with blurring of vision, nausea with a 'livery' feeling and a yellowing of the skin. If this occurs it can take some weeks to clear. It is more likely if a lot of carrot juice is being taken as one glass of carrot juice has around 9,000 I.U. Vitamin A.

Vitamin C: 8-20 grams of sodium or calcium ascorbate daily, dissolved in water and taken orally in three or four divided doses.

Vitamin E: 1 milligram of Micelle E (Bioglan) twice daily (equiv. 150 I.U.).

Formula 4 (Bioglan) [see above]: 1 three times daily.

Selenium: Taken as selenium enriched yeast (1 tablet contains 50 micrograms selenomethionine) aiming for 75-200 micrograms of selenium per day. (Toxic levels he puts at 5 grams per day and says the recommended level is quite safe.)

Thymus Extract: (Bioglan) 1 three times daily.

Enzymes: Digestion Active Enzyme Complex (Bioglan) with each meal. Also Bromelain and Papaine are used sometimes and Apricot Kernels – 5 to 15 kernels daily.

3 Consider daily supplement of Vitamin C, either 10 grams daily or to bowel tolerance.

Food combining

This is like fine tuning – trying to give your digestion combinations of foods that are most easily digested together. Imagine your stomach trying to sort out lobster bisque, beef stroganoff with a side salad, chocolate mousse, all washed down with coffee, then cheese!

To avoid internal warfare, consider the following combining chart:

Food Groups	Primary Proteins	Secondary Pro-teins	Fats	Starches	Melons	Veges.	Sweet Fruits	Sub-Acid Fruits	Acid Fruits
PRIMARY PROTEINS	Good	Poor	Poor	Poor	Poor	Good	Poor	Fair	Good
SECONDARY PROTEINS	Poor	Fair	Poor	Poor	Poor	Good	Poor	Poor	Fair
FATS	Poor	Poor	Good	Fair	Poor	Good	Fair	Fair	Fair
STARCHES	Poor	Poor	Fair	Good	Poor	Good	Fair	Fair	Poor
MELONS	Poor	Poor	Poor	Poor	Good	Poor	Fair	Fair	Poor
VEGETABLES	Good	Good	Good	Good	Poor	Good	Poor	Poor	Poor
SWEET FRUITS	Poor	Poor	Fair	Fair	Fair	Poor	Good	Good	Poor
SUB-ACID FRUITS	Fair	Poor	Fair	Fair	Fair	Poor	Good	Good	Good
ACID FRUITS	Good	Fair	Fair	Poor	Poor	Poor	Poor	Good	Good

Primary Proteins: Almonds, Brazil nuts, Cashew nuts, Hazel nuts, Pine nuts, Pistachios, Walnuts, Pepitas, Sunflower seeds, Sesame seeds, Wheat germ, Lecithin, Soyabean.

Secondary Proteins: Peanuts, Cheese, Eggs, Yogurt, Poultry, Meat, Fish.

Fats: Avocadoes, Oils, Macadamia nuts, Pecan nuts, Coconut, Olives.

Starches: Oats, Rice, Wheat, Corn, Rye, Millet, Buckwheat, Lima beans, Red beans, Pinto beans, Navy beans, Mung beans, Broad beans, Garbanzos, Lentils, Chestnuts, Breadfruit, Jackfruit, Potato, Sweet potato, Jerusalem artichokes, Pumpkin, Taro, Yams.

Melons: Cantaloupe, Watermelon, Honeydew.

Vegetables: Glove artichokes, Fresh sprouts, Beetroot, Carrot, Capsicum, Cucumber, Swedes, Parsley, Brussels sprouts, Cauliflower, Cabbage, Celery, Lettuce, Turnips, Fresh beans, Fresh peas, Zucchini, Chokoes, Marrows, Squash, Broccoli, Asparagus, Eggplant, Silver beet, Spinach, Tomatoes (not with starches), Onions (best cooked).

Sweet Fruits: Bananas, Figs, Custard apples, Monstera deliciosa, Persimmon, All dried fruits.

Sub-Acid Fruits: Mulberry, Raspberry, Blackberry, Blueberry, Grapes, Pears, Apples, Cherries, Apricots, Peaches, Plums, Nectarines, Pawpaws, Mangoes, Guava.

Acid Fruits: Grapefruit, Lemon, Orange, Lime, Mandarin, Pineapple, Strawberry, Kiwifruit (Gooseberry), Passionfruit.

Prepare your food with love and joy, its good stuff!

Food Allergies

Next, be aware of the possibility of food allergies. Common allergenic foods and their alternatives are:

Wheat	Use other grains
Cow's milk	Goat's milk may be suitable
Hen's eggs	Duck eggs may be suitable
Chocolate	Use carob
Shellfish	
Pollen	Avoid if necessary
Tomatoes	

Testing is done via a specialist, or by developing your own sensitivity and awareness. Further discussion of the individualised programme to help identify and avoid allergenic substances occurs later in this chapter. For more details refer to Maureen Minchen's *Food for Thought*.[12]

On Eating Itself:

Wherever possible avoid processed foods that are frozen, canned or dehydrated. Avoid refined foods such as white flour, white rice and margarine. The diet should be low in salt, sugars, fats and proteins. Concentrate on fresh vital foods, primarily vegetables, fruit and grains. Wherever possible, use foods that are in season and grown within a 500 mile radius of your area.

Aim to prepare and eat your food with a sense of joy and the expectation that it will help you back to total health. Take a short time before you eat to be still, relax and be thankful.

Do not over-eat. Do chew your food well – to the consistency of mashed ripe bananas. Digestion begins in the mouth and is aided by a happy, positive disposition. Smile!

Maintenance Diet – Sample Menus We Use

The juices are optional, depending on your situation and preferences.

Summer	Spring/Autumn	Winter
ON ARISING		
Glass of water or	½ water/½ lemon juice or	orange juice
BREAKFAST		
Unlimited amount of one fruit, e.g. water melon, rock melon, etc.	One or more well combined fruits plus 2 tablsp. yoghurt 10-12 almonds 1-2 pieces toast with natural jam Cup herb tea	Porridge – any combination of rolled oats, rye, buckwheat, millet, rice (possibly wheat) or home-made muesli plus 2 tablsp. yoghurt 10-20 almonds 1 tablsp. sultanas 1 stewed apple or equivalent 1-2 pieces toast with natural jam Cup herb tea
MID-MORNING		
Piece of fruit ± almonds ± juice	Piece of fruit ± almonds ± juice	Piece of fruit ± almonds ± juice
MIDDAY		
Juice 2 salad sandwiches with 4-6 vegs. and sprouts, and kelp powder	Juice 2 salad sandwiches with 4-6 vegs. and sprouts, and kelp powder	Juice Soup – veg., miso or vegetable broth. Salad of 4-6 vegs. with bean spread ± bread
MID-AFTERNOON		
Juice	Dandelion coffee ± wholemeal biscuit or cake	Dandelion coffee ± wholemeal biscuit or cake

Summer	Spring/Autumn	Winter
EVENING		
Juice	Juice	Juice
Salad of 4-6 vegs. and sprouts, and sea vegetable, e.g. nori, and tofu or beans	Side salad of 3-4 vegs. and sprouts, followed by dry baked vegs. and rice or pasta dish	50:50 Steamed vegs. and rice or Wholemeal spaghetti and veg./tofu sauce or Veg. pie and rice, etc. Use your flair! Be creative.
BEFORE BED		
Juice	Juice	Juice
May substitute herb teas or equivalent for juices, but latter preferred.		

3 Individual restoration programme

This is a more intense approach. It aims to:

(a) Speed up the process of detoxifying the system.

(b) Hasten development of individual sensitivity to the foods most suitable for you.

(c) Provide the best fuel for restoring your body to health.

It has four phases:

(i) Preparation

A time to gather your information, food and utensils. This is also a time for questioning, understanding and planning. It is a time for making decisions and initiating the change-making process.

Begin moving towards total avoidance of risk factors (see advice on foods to avoid earlier in this chapter). If not already doing so, experiment and become familiar with *meditation*, breathing exercises and enemas, if they are to be used.

In hot weather, 70 per cent to 80 per cent of the diet should be raw, with baked or steamed vegetables in the evening if desired. In cold weather, more cooked food can be taken, e.g. porridge for breakfast.

This is a gentle, introductory time, giving you a chance to

prepare for the changes and benefits. The exact details of what is eaten are not too important at this stage.

The time spent preparing depends on how long it takes to make your decisions and get organised.

(ii) Transition

This is a more intense period. Certainly it has a fasting aspect, without being a fast in the true sense. Fasting on nothing but water appears potentially dangerous for cancer patients and should only be attempted with extremely well experienced medical supervision. I never recommend or suggest it.

This period is intended to help with the principles of detoxifying and cleansing. The idea is to eat only one simple food for a number of days. Several people have recommended that just such a mono-diet can be helpful for cancer patients if carried on for an extended period.

In her book, *The Grape Cure*, Johanna Brandt tells how she used a mono-diet of grapes, backed up by periods on raw foods, as the basis for recovering from her own cancer.[13]

Macrobiotics, the Japanese style of cooking based on their philosophy of balance, recommends that a mono-diet of whole brown rice aids cancer patients to re-balance their system.

Consistently I have found that people who do follow a mono-diet for a short period receive a lot of benefit. They invariably experience what they describe as 'feeling lighter', their taste buds clear and their food begins to taste better. Eating the one thing for a few days certainly works to focus their attention on dietary considerations. It doubles as a good exercise in will-power! Many also find that it does develop the sensitivity that helps them to find their personally appropriate diet. This is a good goal to work towards.

So, in summer, when it is warm and fruit is in season, I suggest that the ideal is ten days eating grapes only. Ten days has been recommended as a good aim but this can be a struggle for some. A minimum of three days is required to see benefit, and I suggest that it is best to set your goal in advance – from three to ten days – and then stick to it.

While doing this, eat as many grapes as you want. Use whatever variety you prefer, but do not mix varieties at one sitting. Drink as little as you feel comfortable with, and then take only pure water or grape juice.

If grapes are not available, then do just three days using half a kilogram of only one fruit at each of three meals, or quarter of a kilogram at each of six meals. Again, drink only pure water or fruit juices, and do not mix different juices and fruits together. Eating only one and a half kilograms of fruit in a day has more of a fasting element than eating unlimited amounts of grapes, but the former is only recommended for three days.

In winter the ideal is ten days on brown rice. The rice should be cooked by the absorption method. One volume of rice plus a half-volume of water is slowly boiled until the water is absorbed. The rice will then be tender. It should be chewed thoroughly - to the consistency of mashed ripe bananas. This may take up to fifty chews per mouthful, so do not be in a hurry! Do eat as much as you want, however, without adding anything else to it.

Again, keeping fluids to a minimum is recommended, and only water should be taken.

Generally the rice is relatively easy, but if you do struggle, some vegetable broth could be added. Exercise should be kept well within your limits and many people find it best to stay close to home, concentrating on the task in hand. If the cold of winter is a problem, warm baths are the best way to warm up thoroughly. Enemas are highly recommended through this transition phase.

Remember this is a time of transition and you may experience some difficulties. Again, appropriate supervision is highly desirable. The more thorough you are the better, but never overlook the need to **keep within your physiological and psychological limits**.

(iii) Regeneration

This is a time to carry on with detoxification and to begin rebuilding a normally functioning system. The emphasis is on fresh, vital and healthy food, as it is a vital and healthy body we want.

This process can be individualised by adding in one food at a time and seeing if it agrees with you or not. Evidence for the role that allergies play in so many diseases is accumulating rapidly and this is a means to identify and avoid them. There is also no doubt that individuals have individual requirements. Do be sensitive to your needs. It requires some will-power to take the time to slowly expand your range of acceptable foods and to say 'No' to things that might disagree. Juices can be added in the same manner.

So, in warm weather, after the transition on grapes or fruit, begin by starting with other fruits. At first stick to one new fruit at each meal. It only takes a few days to try each fruit and then go on to trying combinations. [Refer to the Food Combining Chart in this Chapter] as it is usually best to avoid any suggested poor combinations, e.g. sweet fruit such as banana with an acid fruit such as orange. Then branch out to try the salad vegetables, again being sensitive to anything that does not feel right. Then add grains and other things until a total spectrum emerges.

In cold weather, after a rice transition, add in steamed or baked vegetables first, other grains, then raw vegetables followed by fruits. Follow the scale of cooked grains, cooked vegetables, raw vegetables, cooked fruit, raw fruit. Soon a daily programme will emerge. As an example, these are routines I followed:

Warm Weather Regeneration

AM

7.00 Arise.
a Glass of lukewarm water with 1 tablespoon lemon juice, or b Glass of orange juice (can be 50:50 with water)

7.10 Breathing exercises – preferably bare-footed on grass (glasses removed if normally worn)

7.30 Breakfast: Fruit.
a Any one fruit – I frequently used water melon, or
b Fruit salad with appropriate combinations.

8.00 Caffeine enema.

8.15 Meditate. Ideally one hour.

9.15 Juice. Then,
1 Exercise in open – e.g. walking.
2 Check sprouts, rejuvelac, etc.
3 Smile!

10.30 Juice or piece of fruit or almonds plus herb tea. Then gardening.

PM

12.00 Juice.
Then prepare lunch.

12.30 Lunch. Salad, 4 to 6 salad vegetables, almonds, sprouts.

1.00   Caffeine enema.

1.15   Meditate. Ideally one hour.
        Then free time.

3.00   Juice.
        Then free time.

4.15   Breathing exercises – check you are still smiling!

4.30   Meditate. Ideally one hour.

5.30   Juice.
        Then prepare dinner.

6.00   Dinner. 4 to 6 salad vegetables, sprouts.

6.30   Caffeine enema.

Before bed. Juice or herb tea.
Physically relax on bed and go to sleep with a prayer and/or a positive thought.

Jump out of bed the next morning feeling that little bit better!

This programme could be followed for two weeks, then add in some wholemeal bread for lunch, a vegetable broth for dinner if desired. It is still a fairly strict programme and most people can expect to lose weight. Being lean is an advantage and as long as the weight loss is not excessive it is a good thing. If in doubt, consult your doctor.

Ideally follow this for four weeks before relaxing gradually towards the maintenance diet. If four weeks is a struggle, alternate with two weeks regeneration, two weeks maintenance, and repeat.

Cold weather regeneration

The same basic programme is used but extra cooked food is included with an emphasis on rice. Half the evening meal can be rice, the rest steamed or baked vegetables. Breakfast for the first week can be porridge, for the second week fruit, third week porridge, fourth week fruit again.

Similarly, the winter maintenance diet has a heavier emphasis on grains – particularly if your winters are cold like ours. Then about half the diet should be whole grains.

Grace normally bakes our bread, makes our yoghurt, and

has alfalfa sprouts on the go. We grow virtually all our own vegetables and our orchards should soon provide our fruits.

4 Specific intense diets

As discussed previously, I do not recommend these unless they are
supervised by qualified personnel. My attitude is that a know-
ledgeable doctor should be involved in any such programme.

There are three intensive approaches worth considering. Gerson's diet was the one I followed and feel most comfortable with. It
is extremely intensive and demanding, and only worth considering if you want to make diet a major thing in your life.

Kelley's diet is similar, perhaps not so intense, and I have met
people who claim to have benefited from it.

Macrobiotics offer a whole new approach to diet based on the
philosophy of balance. I have used its principles at times, and
incorporated many of the ideas in with our own. I have reservations concerning the macrobiotic emphasis on cooking nearly all
food for cancer patients although I believe this attitude is changing.

Hopefully these different approaches will be assessed in the
years to come. There is a crying need for meaningful trials to be
carried out to evaluate them.

There has to be an appropriate diet for cancer patients. I believe
that at the moment we can identify the role that diet plays in causing cancer and formulate a range of possibilities in approaching
the role of diet in its treatment. As yet there are no clearcut answers. The final decisions you make must be based on the evidence
available, the advice of those around you, and your own gut
feelings.

Do be warned. Food should be a pleasure as well as our basic
source of sustenance. If you change your diet you can expect some
challenges. Avoid allowing them to become stresses! There is a
great deal to be gained through correct nutrition. Approach this
vast area with a sense of joy and adventure. If you make efforts to
keep your sense of humour, you will receive extra benefits.

A final word on diet

I have always enjoyed ice cream and gelati. I am just about cured of ice cream as it has so many additives, but if a week goes by and I don't have a gelati, I start to get restless. You could say I am addicted. I prefer to say I am happy to indulge in something that pleases me.

There was a time when I felt I was ill enough to concentrate one hundred per cent on diet. I did not have ice cream or gelati for over two years. Now I seek out natural ice cream, or preferably gelati. I recognise that it is probably full of sugar, and perhaps other things I would prefer not to eat.

I know, however, that our maintenance diet at home is close to what we regard as ideal. We grow our own vegetables in rich, well-loved soil. We pick them moments before they come to the table. Soon our orchard will bear our fruit and, in the meantime, virtually all that we do buy in is organically or biodynamically grown.

Grace takes pride in her cooking and prepares our food lovingly, knowing it is our best health insurance. The children reflect the vitality of their food. Rosemary has had a cold for one half of one day in her five years of exuberant life. Her level of awareness of what to eat and why to eat it exceeds that of most adults. She knows ice creams do not agree with her and will not eat them. David aged three-and-a-half, and Peter at two are also showing good signs of discrimination in their choices of food.

But as for me, as I savour my gelati I give thanks for its wonderful taste and swallow it with a smile.

Bon appetit!

Chapter nine

THE CAUSES OF CANCER

It's all in the mind — or is it?

While nutrition and diet are often prominent in their thoughts, ask any cancer patient the question that first went through their mind after they accepted their diagnosis and you will get a common answer: Why me? Why did it happen to me? Why have *I* got this thing? The question is always there. Sometimes it is voiced out loud with anger. Often it remains inside, unexpressed but smouldering with an attendant sense of injustice.

This response is understandable, for there is a popular misconception that the causes of cancer are not known. Therefore patients frequently feel as if they are the victims of a random, vindictive fate. Invariably they find themselves looking around and making comparisons.

'Why not him? Why not old George down the road? He smokes like a chimney, drinks like a fish. Never got a kind word for anyone, never helps anyone, but there he is, eighty years old and still going. Well, I mean I know that I'm no saint, but I sure have been trying to do my best all these years. Why *me!*'

Those who are brave enough to express this vital question out loud often hear: 'I am sorry, we don't really know the causes of cancer'. Or, worse still, they are told: 'It's just one of those things. Bad luck, I suppose'.

Bad luck! Can something as serious as cancer be just 'bad luck'? The whole of the Universe as we know it is governed by Laws. A fundamental one is that for every action there is an equal and opposite reaction. Everything in the physical world is ruled by this Law of cause and effect. The investigative skills of modern technology probe from the smallest atoms to the largest stars and find no exceptions. Can man, the central figure in our Universe, be excluded from similar governing laws? Can cancer really be the product of mere chance?

If the causes of cancer are not identified, then cancer patients are hapless victims of external influences beyond their control. People who feel this to be the case inevitably regard themselves as victims. Such victim-consciousness is probably the most negative emotion in which we can indulge. It allows us to feel as if we had no part in the development of the disease itself; as if the disease just happened and we had nothing to do with it.

Worse, it leaves us feeling helpless, powerless to resist an external force that we can neither understand nor deal with.

To call yourself a cancer 'victim', or to be described as one, conjures up all the worst negative images associated with cancer. Those words, 'cancer victim', should be avoided totally. Cancer itself is not a dirty word, and we should feel free to use it. 'Cancer patient' is fine. Being a patient — someone undergoing treatment — is fine. In another sense, being patient and showing patience, the calm endurance of a situation with attendant perseverance, is a fine attribute. Being a 'victim' is totally inappropriate.

Moreover, the exciting fact is that there is no reason for using the word 'victim'. Most of the causes of cancer can now be identified.

For years it seems as if everyone has been looking for **the** cause: one agent, one food, one chemical, one virus, one anything! Just let there be one thing to blame for the whole problem. It is now obvious that it is not so simple. Cancer has many overlapping causes.

This is the exciting fact. If we are prepared to broaden our horizons and take account of the full spectrum of possibilities we can understand the nature of cancer. There are many factors, not just one, which are involved in producing those final physical symptoms we describe as cancer.

To understand the causes of cancer we must explore the physical, emotional, mental and spiritual realms of man. Not one factor, but many, combine to produce cancer.

Cancer is a multifactorial degenerative disease

Like the camel's back, the body must be labouring under the weight of many burdens before one final straw can break it and allow cancer to develop. This is probably the best news that cancer patients can have! For once the causes of the problem can be identified, it makes it so much easier to take the appropriate action to rectify the situation. If we remove the causes, lift the straws off that broken back, then we have gone a long way towards creating a healing environment. It may be hard, but it can be done.

Virtually all the known causes can be remedied. Cancer is a dynamic process. It is responsive to the influences acting upon it. It is not a one–way, downhill street. It has causes, and those causes produce effects. Remove the disease-producing causes and replace them with health-promoting influences, and health can be recreated.

It is as if there were a set of scales with health and disease producing influences hanging in the balance. When one side prevails - health results; when the other is down – disease. Once the disease scale is down with cancer, it requires an intense effort to tip the balance again. Attending to the sheer physical realities can often require top priority. But, by understanding the disease process, we can set about a rational programme of self-help, based on removing the cancer producing causes and replacing them with health promoting factors.

The starting point is recognising that there is such a process involved, and understanding what set it in motion. Professor Sir Richard Doll, probably the world's leading authority on the causes of cancer, has investigated the physical factors involved.[14] He says that the best current estimates are that, of all cancers (excluding those of the skin), it is reasonable to attribute the cause as follows:

35% to dietary factors
30% to smoking nicotine
10% to infections
7% to sexual excesses
4% to occupational hazards
3% to alcohol
3% to geophysical factors
2% to pollution
1% to medicines and medical procedures
Less than 1% of all cancers are attributable to each of food additives and industrial products.

So, if there were one hundred cancer patients in a random group, we could expect thirty-five of them to be the products of an inappropriate diet.

Exactly which thirty-five may be difficult to determine. We know, however, that a high fat diet is associated with an increased risk of breast cancer. But, for an individual woman in that group who happens to have breast cancer, it is not so easy to say it was caused just by a high fat diet, even if she happened to have been on one. The high fat diet is just one identifiable, and of course very easily rectifiable, factor. However, she may also have been eating a lot of other 'junk' food, drinking alcohol, been emotionally uptight, financially insecure, and so on. The high fat diet may have been the final 'straw' that precipitated her breast cancer. For another woman with the same background burden of risk factors, but without a high fat diet, being a smoker may have been the final straw, or 'trigger factor' that meant she developed cancer, probably lung cancer instead of breast cancer.

Just one trigger factor, such as being a smoker, or having a high fat diet, is not enough on its own to account for the great majority of cancers. I contend that cancer can only occur in a body already weakened by other factors, and not in an otherwise healthy body. These other factors may be physical, psychological and/or spiritual. Some people may have a poor diet as a major precipitating factor. Others may have a large psychological component. The basic idea is that cancer's causes are mostly subtle, usually multiple, frequently synergistic and generally build up over a long period. There may be one final 'trigger factor' that is a more obvious cause than the rest and which precipitated the actual physical symptoms.

Cancer is a chronic, multifactorial, degenerative disease.

The end-point of cancer – the physical symptoms which are a result of the disease – is not so subtle. Once it becomes apparent, it is generally very obvious and often acute. Some cancers, once they do appear, are very fast-moving and potentially life-threatening. The temptation then is to regard them as purely physical problems. There is a tendency to treat only the symptoms rather than the underlying disease, and its collection of causes as well.

In Chapter 8 we looked closely at the physical causes and how to deal with them. Now we turn to examine the other possibilities.

Do not despair! The more causes we identify, the more we can do to overcome them by taking appropriate action. Cancer is a dynamic process. When we replace destructive tendencies with constructive ones, we immediately begin to tip the scales back towards health.

In my experience, psychological factors are important in the causation of most cancers. There is a typical psychological profile which occurs in over 95 per cent of all the many cancer patients with whom I have discussed their disease. (Through my work with the Melbourne Cancer Support Group and through seminars conducted in all the Australian States, this number now exceeds one thousand.) This profile was first expounded by Dr E. Evans in 1926! It has gained increasing attention over the last few years, especially in the work of Dr Lawrence Le Shan[15] and that of Dr Carl Simonton and Stephanie Matthews[16].

This increase in attention is important for, if the psychological factor is identified and treated appropriately, then a major driving force that has been keeping the cancer going is immediately removed.

Most cancer patients recognise this psychological profile. For some it comes as a shock to hear their basic life history so accurately recounted.

1   Childhood stress

In childhood, a cluster of stresses build up over a period of time. The stresses often relate to the child's interaction with their parents or peers, the prime influences acting in their life at this time. The stress may come from parents who are physically violent or from those who are emotionally non-expressive or abusive. It may be the product of the child feeling they have little worth because they do not feel loved or get little encouragement in their endeavours.

2   Climactic event

There comes one final incident which, again, is like the final straw that breaks the camel's back. Usually occurring around seven to nine years of age, this event seems almost unbearable. The child cries enough. They know that they cannot endure that type of stress any more. Something has to give, and it is them. Something snaps inside, the shutters go down. No longer can the child react in a free, uncomplicated manner.

3 Premeditated pattern of behaviour

The child realises it needs some defence pattern to cope with the situation. They decide to adopt a rigid pattern of behaviour in response to stress. By doing so the stress becomes manageable; life becomes tolerable again.

Very frequently, in cancer patients, this rigid pattern of behaviour revolves around attempting to be as other people want them to be, rather than as they personally feel they should be. This commonly leads them on to try to please other people, to do as others would want them to. There is often an overtone of passive subservience. They are not the types to become aggressive or anti-social. They want to be liked.

So cancer patients are frequently 'nice' people. When diagnosed, their friends often say, 'Why her? She's so nice, always trying to help other people. Why her? Why not that old creep George down the road?'

The fact is, of course, that trying to please other people is a fine ideal. It is the motivation behind it, however, that creates problems for cancer patients. For them, this begins as a conscious means of coping, a defence mechanism, not a pure motivation. It is taken up as a premeditated defence mechanism and means they become reliant on factors outside themselves, outside their control, for their fundamental happiness and sense of worth.

4 Rigid response becomes automatic

This conscious effort to be a particular type of person is soon repeated so often that it becomes an automatic response. Now all stress is handled in the same basic, rigid way.

As this involves putting other people first, this pattern works well and they are liked and usually successful. They frequently seek out positions where they can gain their gratification through the approval of others. It is not easy for them to do things based simply on their merits and to be satisfied by them. They find it difficult to develop a good self-image, and frequently rely on others for their own self-esteem. This need for outside approval is very real, if not always consciously expressed. Outwardly, their rigid pattern of behaviour can produce a confident and assured air, but all the time they are seeking to cover this lack of self-esteem. Deep down, there can lurk a marked lack of self-confidence with a tendency towards self-negation, almost self-destruction. Deeply bottled inside is the feeling that all is not well. True reactions, emotions especially, are often suppressed. There is a continual effort to block out basic feelings. It is like trying to push the truth from the conscious awareness, like trying to keep the lid on a constantly bubbling pressure cooker.

Inner tension is established and maintained. There is a limited range of responses possible when it comes to dealing with stress.

5   Another major climactic stress

In later life, another cluster of stresses is followed by one major event which changes the patient's whole life circumstances. For example, we see this happening with people who have put all their emotional security into one relationship. Then if that relationship fails through death or separation, the sense of loss can be profound indeed. This can involve relationships with parents, lovers, spouses or even with a devoted mother whose children leave home. The same effect can occur when a 'workaholic' retires or is put out of work. Suddenly there is no outlet. Their whole life pattern is upset. Financial difficulties followed by a foreclosure may be enough to tip the balance for some people.

6   Inability to cope

This change in life circumstances threatens the person's very source of self-worth and purpose. There seems to be no way their rigid pattern of behaviour can deal with it. Their very life has been undermined. The person feels to be a victim of circumstances beyond their control and they can see no answer to this new situation. They feel as if life has dealt them a bitter blow, often one which they half expected to occur. Life no longer has any meaning for them. Because they do not feel that they can change their way of coping, they can see no viable future.

7   Feelings of hopelessness

Faced with an unsolvable problem, a feeling of hopelessness develops. It is as if they feel trapped by external circumstances and are unable to do anything in response.

On the outside, however, their rigid pattern of behaviour keeps them going. Often they carry on with their rigid, cheery, helpful front. They are often unable to express their loss, and outsiders often remark how well they seem to be coping, how little they have changed despite their adversity.

Inside, they feel shattered.

8 Body mirrors hopelessness

This inner sense of hopelessness is soon mirrored by the body itself. It is as if the body, too, gives up. It is as if the body also loses the will to live, it loses the ability to defend itself. The effect is a great drop in the effectiveness of the body's own physical defences, the immune system.

Again, this concept ties in so well with the idea that cancer involves a basic fault in the body's own natural function. It is as if this stress is so major that the body is laid open to having cancer, a self-destructive disease, develop. Another straw, another major cause, becomes apparent.

In my experience most cancer patients can see this scenario in their life. Most recognise a climactic stressful event three months to two years before their symptoms first appeared. The most common interval, by far, for the people I have worked with, has been eighteen months. It is as if it takes this long for the body to produce the external symptoms of that internal state.

The key factor here, the key problem, is the inability to cope with major stress. Now, during their lives most people will have similar events involving such major stress. These stresses are an inevitable part of life. Dr Thomas Holmes has done interesting work in this area and attempted to quantify the effects of life-changing stress on our lives. He has developed a Social Readjustment Rating Scale, published in *Getting Well Again* by O. C. Simonton and S. Matthews, which puts a relative figure on various potentially stressful events.[17] Starting with loss of a spouse at 100 points, it goes through a range of negative and, significantly, positive life situations that all *can* affect our well-being. (Coping with personal success can be just as potentially stressful as reversals.)

Social Readjustment Rating Scale

Event	Value
Death of spouse	100
Divorce	73
Marital separation	65
Jail term	63
Death of close family member	63
Personal injury or illness	53
Marriage	50
Fired from work	47
Marital reconciliation	45
Retirement	45
Change in family member's health	44
Pregnancy	40
Sex difficulties	39
Addition to family	39
Business readjustment	39
Change in financial status	38
Death of close friend	37
Change to different line of work	36
Change in number of marital arguments	36
Mortgage or loan over $10,000	31
Foreclosure of mortgage or loan	30
Change in work responsibilities	29
Son or daughter leaving home	29
Trouble with in-laws	29
Outstanding personal achievement	28
Spouse begins or stops work	26
Starting or finishing school	26
Change in living conditions	25
Revision of personal habits	24
Trouble with boss	23
Change in work hours, conditions	20
Change in residence	20
Change in schools	20
Change in recreational habits	19
Change in church activities	19
Change in social activities	18
Mortgage or loan under $10,000	17
Change in sleeping habits	16
Change in number of family gatherings	15
Change in eating habits	15
Vacation	13
Christmas season	12
Minor violation of the law	11

A score of over 300 from the table in any one year produced a 50 per cent chance of developing illness, while a score of under 200 produced less than 10 per cent of risk. This demonstrates that direct link between stress and illness: the more stress, the more illness produced.

The emphasis with all these factors is the change they produce in our life circumstances. What is at issue, then, is the ability to adapt to change. The fact is that we commonly seek to preserve the *status quo* and find change a hard thing to make.

Most people, however, do pass through such periods of stress, are able to effect changes, and life goes on. While major clusters of stress may produce a temporary setback, even related physical disease, most people do bound back. They have some means of coping or are able to adapt to their new circumstances. They do not feel hopeless for any lasting period. We need to remember the difference between a challenge and a stress.

For cancer patients, it is not so much the nature of the challenge that is such a problem, as their reaction to it. This is most important. Everyone is subjected to challenges. Everyone is likely to be faced with some major life-changing events during their lifetime. Whether it be the death of a loved one, the need to change jobs, move to a new city, whatever, such events are inevitable. Certainly many of the lesser challenges in our lives actually give it zest and flavour. Many challenges work to extend and develop us and life would be pretty dull without them.

The problem for cancer patients, then, is this inability to cope with a major challenge, particularly when it involves a fundamental change in their life. The inability to react appropriately and find release from the situation produces the changes in body chemistry we know as stress. This in turn lowers the immune system and so adds a significant factor to the list of causes of cancer. The more I talk with individual patients and groups, the more I am convinced of the importance of this factor.

Being able to recognise this in their nature is a great asset for a cancer patient. By accepting that this did contribute to their situation, they can make a great deal more sense of it. It is then relatively simple, in principle at least, to learn to cope with these psychological aspects of stress. By dealing with it appropriately, patients can contribute greatly to their own well-being and return to health. We shall explore in more detail the means available to do this in the next chapter.

Finally, however, having considered the physical and psychological causes of cancer, we need to go one step further. We need to be brave enough to ask, 'Why me?' once more.

Why do some people have this cancer profile, not others? Why do only some people find themselves in those complex childhood situations that lead on to particular attitudes and a pattern of behaviour which, in turn, predisposes them to cancer? Why are some people drawn to smoke, to eat potentially harmful foods, to work in dangerous environments, and as a consequence be faced with disease?

Unless we can answer these harder questions, we will remain unsatisfied and still be tempted to wallow in victim-consciousness. Again, is it just chance that these circumstances develop? Surely not! We are now faced with a basic philosophical question that must be tackled.

I consider myself fortunate. Right from the time my cancer was first diagnosed, I recognised that there was a spiritual thread running through and connecting all the events in my life. Moreover, I felt that I had been living with a disharmony between my inner spiritual attitudes and my outer physical actions. There was conflict between what I felt I should do and what I actually did. While I was not doing anything illegal, even dishonest, to other people, I felt I was not being true to my own inner aspirations. I felt that this disharmony was another major factor in the development of my cancer and so I had another avenue to work with in getting well. This attitude provided me with a basic stimulus and *raison d'être* for seeking harmony in my spiritual, psychological and physical nature. I saw the three as interwoven and interdependent. Because I could see the interrelatedness of my past actions and present circumstances, and felt confident that the law of cause and effect did govern my life, I felt confident that justice would prevail. If I could make the necessary changes and find the right techniques, health should be reattainable.

Now it is relatively easy to talk of psychological and physical things. The issues are relatively straightforward and not too emotionally charged. It is not so easy with things spiritual. However, knowing the important stimulus it was to me, and having seen so many others gain strength and direction from their own spiritual endeavour, I feel it appropriate to delve into these deeper areas.

I hesitate for just a moment as I do not want to be labelled, nor do I want to run the risk of having good, straightforward techniques like *meditation* labelled. All these techniques do stand independently in their own right and are quite free of spiritual bias. They can all be judged on their own merits.

At the same time I feel that any life is rather facile without some spiritual loading. Most cancer patients are interested – in fact, they are often preoccupied – with the quest for a basic spiritual reality. Many people do favour their life with spiritual concerns and it is appropriate to recognise this. Being raised in the Church of England I consider myself, now more than ever, very much a Christian. Perhaps the answers I have found and accept, and which remain open to change, are not the orthodox Christian ones. There is no doubt I have been influenced by the other major world religions. I like to talk of my attitudes as a means to provoke discussion in this vital area.

So, why should any person be placed in that combination of conditions that eventually leads to cancer? While people do seem to learn best and develop most through adversity, is it really necessary to go through cancer? And why should young children get it? There must be some reason why.

It is really a clear-cut, basic choice. There is either order or there is not. Either we have to say life is meaningless and harsh in the extreme as no Loving God could allow such things, or we say there is some order, some reason for it, some logic behind it all. I confess to not being able to make sense of what I see happening around me just on face value. Why do some people get it easy, others apparently hard?

I have an undying faith in the basic structured order of the Universe. There has to be an explanation. The only one that satisfies me is provided by the Eastern philosophy of karma and reincarnation, the spiritual laws of cause and effect.

Karma is a concept which says that every action we make produces an equal reaction. As we sow, so we reap. Good action, good consequences, and the opportunity to benefit by them; bad action, bad consequences, and the need to face those consequences and learn to get it right. We can certainly see this principle operating in current life circumstances. Most of our current situation is the product of events we can easily identify. But it is often difficult to see justice or order in all of our own life patterns and certainly it is easy to judge some others harshly. Still others seem to face impossibly difficult odds in life, while on the surface they appear blameless. I am drawn, therefore, to widen my frame of reference to include the concept of reincarnation. If we do pass from life to life and carry over basic traits and blemishes, it makes sense of many seemingly inexplicable events. The child genius, the congenital birth defects, the hopelessly poor, the uncaring rich, all assume explainable stations in life.

For me, these concepts provide a framework into which I can comfortably fit and feel confident working in. Seeing successive lifetimes as opportunities for spiritual evolution provides a reason to strive for ethical conduct in all situations. It also means that no effort is wasted. Every attempt we make to reach a greater degree of harmony in our lives will eventually bear fruit. Any effort, be it in the physical, psychological or spiritual realm, if made with a positive, harmonious motivation, will be to our benefit.

Recognising this spiritual thread to life and its ongoing nature was a great comfort for me as I battled the odds. It helped me to understand my situation, even if I could not relate my present predicament to definite events of a previous lifetime. Also, it made me feel the efforts of attempting to get well were worthwhile. Death lost its sting as final arbitrator. If life went on and my attitudes and actions had effects on my future circumstances, it meant I should try 100 per cent in every situation. Anything more I could not do, but anything less would be totally inappropriate. Finally I had to realise that I had to do my 100 per cent and then be prepared to let the results take care of themselves. I had to learn the need to avoid being attached to the results of my actions and not to view them as win or lose situations.

Similarly, I came to recognise and accept that I was truly responsible for my own condition. It is relatively easy to accept our role in disease through our patterns of eating and thinking and the environment in which we live. I feel it even more satisfying to see disease as an opportunity for soul growth through learning and endeavour. Our soul has put us in this position to test our reactions and gives us the opportunity to learn the lessons we need in a very intense way. We never get more than we have the potential to handle! Remember the people who say, 'Cancer has taught me so much; much more than I could have learned without it'.

It is vital to recognise in all this that cancer is a dynamic situation. It is good to recognise what causes you can in your own life as then you can act, make changes and get well again. This thinking gives a rationale for a total approach for treatment.

On the physical level, the actual symptoms should certainly not be neglected. Appropriate direct therapy should be considered for them. However, do not overlook that the lumps and bumps are only symptoms. Do not forget to tackle the underlying causes. Again, on the physical level, this means removing toxic inputs wherever possible. It makes good sense at least to have an organic maintenance diet and to avoid any sources of pollution. It also makes sense to utilise any treatment that increases the body's natural defences.

Psychologically, the big need is to change. If we recognise that a particular pattern has aided in creating the disease, then obviously a new pattern is required. Changing to that new pattern can be done through conscious action based on the desire to get better. However, often it will just flow on as a result of the disease itself. The disease creates the excuse for change. It produces a new situation or insight that allows the patient the space to change their rigid patterns.

Hope is the key here. It may come from within with a change of attitude or be built by inspiration from without. Once that hope is revived, then the rebuilding process is under way. The attitude becomes positive and pro-life. The sense of being a victim gives way to a feeling of being responsible and in control.

Many find that they no longer feel guilt about their past. Their new perspective sheds fresh light and allows them to seek forgiveness for errors of the past. Now they feel free to concentrate on building a new future, to concentrate on loving life and all around them.

One step leads on to the next, and the physical condition soon reflects this improvement. While there may be ups and downs, the healing process gathers momentum. Frequently, passive *meditation* takes the bumps out of this path. Having benefits on all levels of our being, it both smooths out and intensifies the healing.

For many people, the end result is a health that is described as 'weller than well'. Having recovered from such an illness, they have a new zest for life. Just getting well from cancer is cause enough for a boost in self-esteem. Add to this all that is learned along the way, and people frequently portray a new confidence and a quiet but genuine regard for themselves. The joy they feel enhances their own lives and infuses joy into those with whom they come in contact. *It is a process of self-discovery and self-fulfilment.*

Chapter ten

DEALING WITH STRESS

With knowledge and love

As we go on to consider how to deal with the major area of stress, we need to begin by examining what it is that turns a challenge into a stress. Why is it that in the lives of some of us challenges are left unresolved, or we can find no appropriate response to them and so become locked into stress? Why are we unable to accept challenges, and why can't we accept our responses to them as being satisfactory and reasonable? *Why* do we get stressed?

Challenges can be positive or negative in nature. Many challenges we accept as opportunities to use our skills and talents, to extend ourselves, to create, to assist – to be positive. These are the challenges that add to and enhance our lives. It should be realised that they can produce inner tension, but that this is a creative, positive, non-harmful tension.

So what is the factor that makes challenges negative and creates stress? At the root of *all* the many different types of stress, I contend that there is one basic problem – *fear*.

Fear is a painful emotion caused by impending danger, a state of alarm. In the natural flow of events, fear stimulates the fight-or-flight response. It should precede appropriate action but, if it does not, and the alarm signals keep sounding, it produces stress. In days gone by, the causes of fear were immediate, obvious and physical. In current times they are chronic, subtle and multi-faceted.

So, to treat stress we need to consider treating fear. This we can do admirably. On a mental level, *knowledge* dispels fear, while, on an emotional level, *love* works every time. While love is a much bandied about word these days, do not be fooled by the simplicity of this. Love is the appropriate response to fear each and every time it occurs. It works, one hundred per cent, every time.

Let us begin, however, by seeking to *understand* the fear in our lives. The immediate fears are usually obvious, but what of the old, deep-seated, nagging ones? From the outset, there is no need to feel any guilt in looking back over difficult areas in our lives. We seek to understand the circumstances in our lives that have contributed to our present situation. By accepting disease as a dynamic cause/effect situation, we can also accept responsibility for our own situation and work back to health. Having recognised our role in creating our present situation, and accepting the present, we can look forward to our role in the future.

This is a good area in which to identify problems as once they are identified they are easy to treat. There are good techniques readily available. Again, the final indicator is that when we are free of stress we will be free of tension. Relaxed in body, mind and spirit.

So, looking back at the cancer profile, what type of fears are they that cause stress in children? Some will have fears of physical assault, but more often the fears are of psychological assault. 'If I don't do what I'm told, or expected, Mummy and Daddy won't like me any more. Worse, they might not love me.' A child lives and grows by love. It has a deep inner urge to love and be loved. To *not* be loved, to be rejected is an enormous cause of fear in any child.

Now, as I see it, children are incredibly adaptable and malleable. They will accept almost any difficulties and their native love of life and eagerness to experience it will carry them on – that is, until they strike rejection or the lack of love. If this is accompanied by a major crisis, their whole world can be jeopardised. While suicide is one of the highest forms of teenage death in America, most children do manage to adapt. Others become anti-social, difficult people. The cancer types, however, try to win affection, to do things that make them worthy of love. They develop a rigid pattern of behaviour as a defence reaction.

As adults, they carry with them the fear of rejection as an ongoing, deep-seated one. It can undermine their relationships, limiting their range of emotions with family and friends. They are always looking for something, seeking the thing they sense missing from their lives. Frequently, it will be displaced to form new fears, as their self-esteem can only be gained through the approval of others. Status may become important, whether it be as a successful owner of material wealth, as a provider or a parent.

With this deep inner tension always present, if mostly controlled, a major crisis can produce insurmountable stress. A change in life circumstances can lead to their worst fears being realised. For when the means of handling this seemingly lifelong pain of a fear of rejection, is taken away, what hope is left? With no apparent solution to the problem, the will to live crumbles.

Now, there is no physical reason why a person in such a state should die. But, as the mind gives up, the body follows suit. The effect the mind can play in this way is graphically demonstrated by the Australian Aborigines. If a member of a tribe, which is always a close-knit unit, transgresses a major tribal law, he may be subjected to the ultimate punishment – pointing the bone. Amidst much ceremony the offender is told what he has done, how his action makes him worthless in the eyes of the tribe and why he should die. Then the medicine man of the tribe symbolically points the bone at him. The effect is electric. A man who saw it happen described it to me. The offender was a young man in perfect health. As soon as the bone was pointed at him, however, his whole body began to stiffen and become rigid. No amount of the white man's aid could reverse the process. He developed a faraway, hopeless look and refused all food. Within a few days this apparently healthy man had collapsed and died.

There is another recent case where an Aboriginal was saved after having the bone pointed. An astute white man announced to the dying man that he, too, was a medicine man of high degree and that he could remove the evil force from him. Amidst much ceremony, and a little conjuring, he produced an object from the man's abdomen and ritually destroyed it. The Aboriginal began to recover immediately and did so completely!

Cancer patients are often going through a similar process. Now, I am not saying this psychological component is *the* cause of cancer, but I am sure that it occurs too frequently to be ignored. It is another major contributing factor.

For many then, once the cancer is actually diagnosed, a truly hopeless situation will exist. Hope is based on desire and expectation. Often the cancer patient has already lost the desire to live and now the diagnosis gives him the opportunity to not expect to live. A rather blunt friend, a fellow cancer patient, once described cancer as a socially acceptable form of suicide for people who found themselves in an intolerable position.

I can hear people yelling in protest, 'It's not me! That's not me!' However, it is usually the families, not the patients, who protest most. Many patients recognise the sequence readily, are relieved to understand what is going on and happy to set about correcting the situation. Hope becomes the starting point. To re-create hope we need to bolster the desire to live and the expectation that a continuation of life is possible.

The desire or will to live can often be rekindled by the diagnosis! Having cancer can change a person's life dramatically and totally. Suddenly they become the centre of attention. Friends and family rally, work may be avoided, a ready excuse is available for that long put off holiday, all manner of new possibilities present.

Some patients become very good at it – at being patients. They may have a flourishing victim consciousness, but under all the attention they rally. Life becomes enjoyable and worth living again, and the body responds to this new surge. Many then find new ways of coping and do get back to leading healthy lives again. Some then come to that difficult point where they are getting so well that friends no longer call, the family returns to its own normal pursuits, and the need to work re-emerges. A difficult choice: to be sick and happy; or well and miserable. It would be funny if it was not real. It would be foolish to oversimplify the complexity of this problem, but, so frequently, psychological trauma is a major consideration for cancer patients.

The cry of anguish that creates disease is a cry for love. It is a genuine need that should be met. Love is the appropriate response and it works one hundred per cent every time.

In my experience, emotional factors do play a major role in cancer. Cancer patients are frequently emotionally tight. They prefer to keep their emotions to themselves and have difficulty in expressing them even if they want to. It has taken me years to feel comfortable telling people how I feel about them, particularly if I want to express my feelings of love.

When we recollect the sequence of: *challenge – bodily reaction –*

physical action – release and the psychological profile involved in cancer, we see that the challenge in that profile is frequently emotionally based. The fear that turns it into a stress is usually one of not being loved, of being rejected, or of being emotionally hurt.

For cancer patients it is most frequently emotional challenges that produce the bodily reaction of changes in body chemistry. For them, there often seems to be no adequate action that can be taken to resolve their situation and so gain release.

Emotional fear fixes them in a state of *altered body chemistry*. The contention is that this can be so profound as to reduce their immune response. Then, when a cancer begins – as might be prompted by a high-fat diet, cigarette smoking, some bodily malfunction, or whatever – the body no longer cares, it no longer recognises it has a problem. It allows the cancer to develop and life-threatening symptoms can follow.

This being so, it is vital for cancer patients to work on their emotions, too – to 'let go' emotionally, to heal the emotions as well as the body. Most people enjoy this part of it, once they get going! Everyone wants to feel love in their life and feel capable of giving it freely.

It starts on a physical level, and touch is most important. Through touch we can communicate so much, often far more than we can with words. How often have you been to a doctor who did not do anything special, but you still came away feeling better? He had a good 'touch'. It's real. People who care, convey it by touch. Many Western people have been trained that it is 'sissy', or worse, to touch. It is not. It is a good thing to do. Encourage it amongst your family and close friends at least. An arm around the shoulder, a squeeze of an arm, a hug, it all works wonders.

I love seeing visitors at our place inter-acting with Rosemary. At five she is a very touching person. If she goes for a walk she likes to hold hands. She puts one hundred per cent into her cuddles. Many friends react awkwardly. You can see they enjoy this natural show of affection, but is it all right to be doing it? Usually they decide it is, lose their stiffness and smile a lot.

Massage has the same valuable quality of touch. Not only does it release physical tension, but a good masseur conveys that love flow and helps to release emotional energy. This is nothing erotic;

it is indeed unfortunate that massage has other connotations these days. Good massage is indeed sensual, being a thing involving the sense of touch, but not sexual. True massage is a wonderful healing medium. It is easy to do and highly recommended amongst couples and families.

Smiling, and especially laughter, are probably the best emotional release valves we have. When all else fails, laugh! Again, this is not flippant; you should seek out opportunities to laugh and enjoy doing something that does you so much good.

On the psychological level, hope is the prime motivator. Hope, remember, is based on desire and expectation. Desire is adversely affected by stress, which is based on fear. For most cancer patients, that fear is an emotional fear. The simple antidote for emotional fear is love. So, desire to experience love in your life. Let love be your goal. Then you will experience peace of mind instead of conflict.

In reality the choice is yours in every situation. You can choose to experience conflict or peace. When you make the effort to choose peace, your life becomes harmonious. It is that simple. You need to fix in your mind, affirm regularly, this desire to experience peace of mind as your reality.

So, let us consider how this applies to relationships. With whom do you have the most important relationship – your wife, son, mother, or none of these? It is yourself! We all know that old maxim, 'Love thy neighbour as thy self'. Yet we seem preoccupied with the first half of the saying. Everyone wants to be seen as loving and helping their fellows, but they overlook the '. . . as thy self' bit. This is the really vital part. If you do not have a good relationship with yourself, if you do not feel good about yourself, if you do not love yourself, you can never relate openly or love honestly. You will be looking to other relationships to cover up your own seeming inadequacies, or seeking out people who show you in a good light. Relationships will be clouded by loadings you impose on them. Only when you love yourself can you love another. This is not love in an egotistical sense, nor is it any other false emotion. It is a basic human right. You should love yourself.

'Why should I?' you say. There is every reason. 'But am I not fat? Haven't I got a crooked nose? My hair is not what I'd like and, besides, haven't I got cancer?'.

You have a body that is so complex, so intricate, delicate and wonderful that if you look at it, really look at it, you cannot fail to be impressed. Your heart pumps 100,000 times each and every day. Can you imagine that? No mechanical pump could come close to doing it. Especially without regular overhauls and repairs, and yet you do. No one else does it for you. Your body does it, regularly, automatically.

Think again. There was a time when you were just two cells: one from your mother, one from your father. They merged, became one, and then began dividing again. From those two cells, just two, your whole body has been created. In the process you have mirrored evolution. In the warmth of your mother you passed from being two cells through stages like a protoplasm, fish, reptile, animal, to man. You have this incredible, creative, inner force that has created the body which is exactly right for you at this moment in your evolution. Sometimes you may wonder at that, but you are in the right shape, in the right place, to learn the right lessons and experience what is right for you *now*. You produced it all!

This same creative force maintains your health. It can heal broken bones with ease. Given the right conditions, it can heal or create anything.

Those right conditions begin with love of self. That love is innate, a part of our natural being. Children show it perfectly, adults often cloud it through fear. It grows, however, with reverent awe as the true wonder of the body and soul are realised. If you have difficulty with this, I suggest you have another of those clearcut choices. You either love yourself or you do not. It is a simple, basic choice.

If you want to reinforce that love, or come to feel it, meditate and contemplate it. Think of yourself. Think of the workings of your body, emotions, mind and Soul. As you contemplate this, you may well become aware how your outer realities are temporary ones. Your body, your personality, your environment are all changing so rapidly and frequently. But in the stillness you may become aware of something more permanent, more stable, more meaningful. This, your inner core, your true self, is what you need to recognise and love. Then you will be able to accept that you have limitations; everyone has those external limits. Accept that you have strengths. Think how you can put them to good use.

Come to the point where you can accept totally that 'Yes, I am worthy of my Love. Because I have this inner core which is pure and true and unviolable'.

Be prepared to admit your outer weaknesses in a non-defensive, non-aggressive, open way. Be prepared to put your strengths forward and to make good with them. Know that you have that inner core which is perfect.

You will find that, when you do, your relationships with others will improve dramatically. You will be able to be more open and responsive, and everyone will benefit. You can use some simple techniques to aid this process. Seek to praise, not criticise. I had a graphic lesson in this. Having been an athlete, I was always conscious of 'style' in running. I enjoyed watching others who had it and tried to develop it myself. It gave me joy to aim to learn to run with style and the more I worked at it the faster I went. Following my amputation, I then spent a lot of time trying to move on crutches with 'style'. Sounds funny, I suppose, but I tried to move fluidly and easily. I never told anyone about my 'training'. One day a young man quite unknown to me came up and said, 'It is a pleasure to watch you move. You look as if you are just floating along', and left. Nobody else before or since has ever commented. Most people simply ask me what happened and why I don't wear an artificial leg. While I have always felt comfortable with crutches and obviously prefer to use them, that single remark, said with genuine feeling, always sticks in my mind and reinforces my feeling good about them. The old saying, 'A word of praise is worth a thousand of criticism', is so true. You can make someone else's day by seeking out what it is that deserves praise. A single, well-placed, genuinely felt word can have someone else smiling for a long time.

Thank people for what they do for you. You probably take for granted that someone who is helping you knows how helpful they are being. They probably don't. Tell them. It reinforces their kindness and leaves them in no doubt. If they are trying to help and not succeeding, tell them. Give them the opportunity to do something constructive, and show you care.

If you want love to come into your life, it must also flow out. Love is cyclical – it cannot flow in one dead-end direction. Seek ways to give your love to others. This is most important. It gets patients' whole rhythm moving when they start to give to others. Some do this by simple prayer, others by communal service. Some practise tithing and, well – Jazzer, he just gave everything.

The more Jazzer gives the more he receives. He reckons if he really needed a Rolls Royce someone would give it to him. Not that he wants one, but if he really *needed* it, he knows it would be there. Jazzer constantly gives to others. There was a time when he was doing a promotion for singer Johnny Farnham. His wife was quite a fan and had just bought his latest album. One Friday night the record was playing when an eight-year-old girl from up the street visited. She, too, loved the music, and danced and sang as it played. Before his wife's disbelieving eyes, Jazzer took the record off the player and gave it to the little girl. Next Monday, Jazzer duly arrived at work to find on his desk an autographed copy of the same L.P. sent by Johnny in appreciation for his help.

Another time Jazzer learned of a lady thousands of miles away who was in financial trouble. He arranged through his firm's accountants to have twenty dollars sent to her in a way that made it untraceable. At that time many people were being laid off in his office, and all the remainder were concerned about their jobs. One day Jazzer was delivering copy to another large agency when the manager called him in for a friendly chat. The manager of the firm for whom Jazzer worked happened to drop some material in at this time and saw him talking to the opposition's head.

On returning to his office, Jazzer was summoned to the manager's office. 'Now, Jazzer, I know we have been laying quite a few people off, but you are one we want to keep. I know you have been looking around, but we'd like you to stay. As a token of the regard we hold you in, there will be an extra $20 in your pay packet as of now.' Give and you will receive.

Of course, *meditation* is also a very valuable tool for improving emotional well-being. Again, passive *meditation* leads to acceptance of self which enables us to be more open with others.

Be aware, also, that the technique of being relaxed under stress leads to defusing many potentially difficult situations. If you feel an emotional confrontation developing, make sure you keep physically relaxed. I often reinforce this by feeling relaxation flow through me as I breathe out. A gentle sigh at the same time accentuates the feeling of relaxation. Some like to say 'relax' as they breathe out. It is amazing how well this will defuse a situation where someone else is getting agitated. Realising that their rage, anger, or whatever negative emotion, is theirs and does not have to be yours, helps even more. You *can* accept their negative emotion to experience as your own, or you can seek peace and reinforce it with relaxation.

I am amazed at how this works with animals in my veterinary surgery. When I first graduated, I was busy and not very sensitive to the animals' needs. We used to have regular brawls trying to control aggressive animals. Now we find that by concentrating on not showing – better, not feeling – fear and spending time with the animals and communicating with them by talking and touching, we very rarely have any problems.

There is a final technique which is a valuable aid in dealing with difficult relationships. We all have been involved in relationships in the past that have not been as we would have liked. This is quite normal but often we get so enmeshed that the situation seems irretrievable and we can see no way around it. Such relationships can often be a constant sore point and a cause for chronic emotional stress. We need a way to let them go.

This can be done by using another meditation technique, which starts with:

Relaxation. Just as you normally would, take up a slightly uncomfortable position, preferably sitting or squatting, and go through the standard relaxation.

Visualise the person you are considering. It is all right to just concentrate on them, but try to build up as clear an image of them in your mind as you can, as if they were sitting in front of you and you were looking directly at them.

Then use these four phrases, repeating *each* one silently to yourself, over and over, until you can say it with conviction, before going on to the next:

> I forgive you.
>
> Please forgive me
>
> I thank you.
>
> I bless you.

As you begin this exercise, you will find that it takes an effort to concentrate on the person's image *and* the repetition of 'I forgive you, I forgive you'. Then you will probably begin to think of all the good reasons why you should *not* forgive them.

'Forgive *them!* I have every reason to hate that person!' you may think. Every reason, except that hate affects *you* more than anyone else! As you dwell on it more, a wider, healthier perspective will come.

As you keep repeating the phrase, you enter into meditating on why you should forgive them. Think of all the reasons they are like they are, why they did what they did. You will find yourself slipping over into contemplation and a new insight developing. As you continue you *will* reach the point where, with conviction, you can say, 'I forgive you!' I found 'Please forgive me?' was the hard one; however, the more I did this exercise the more I came to realise my role in all the problems. If I had behaved differently, the whole situation would have developed in a better, more harmonious way.

'I thank you' was sometimes something of a test, too. Thanking someone for putting you through a hard time that finally taught you so much demands a perspective of forgiveness and acceptance. This exercise develops a great understanding of life and relationships in general.

'I bless you' is easy after the first three have reached the point of conviction. It is a release, a letting go. At that point you recognise the worth in the other person. While you may agree to differ on points of view, you are now free to go your independent ways without any negative attachments.

I found it good to start this exercise with easy things, like the man who cut you off while driving home, the lady who stood on your toe, or the shop assistant who was so difficult. It is a good thing to do as a regular exercise – once a day for a while. I used to choose someone that I had met during each day and practise it 'with' them. Soon I found the whole thing happening automatically as any incident occurred. If a difficulty with a relationship looked like developing, it was as if those four little phrases whizzed around in my head, defusing the situation even before it developed. Then I worked on the hard relationships, the cluttered old ones from time gone by. The effect was considerable. I really felt freed of old attachments.

Alcoholics Anonymous takes this idea further and suggests that reformed alcoholics should make restitution to people they have harmed. They recommend actually fronting such people, apologising and doing all they can to physically make good any loss they caused. I do not think it is necessary for cancer patients using this method to go that far unless they want to. However, I know it works, for there was one particular person that I had been involved with in a difficult way and had not felt comfortable with since. I practised the technique until I really could genuinely say those four statements. When I then called on the person, the atmosphere between us was totally different to the usual tension. We fell easily into an extended talk, discussing all our old problems, and both left feeling lighter and happier. It amazed me that the whole nature of that relationship was balanced by that exercise. Many of the cancer patients in our group have found it works for them and I recommend it highly.

All efforts are rewarded, and giving more love to others brings more back into your own life. Love is the greatest healer.

Inspiration can also help remotivate people. This may come through an individual, a group, the church, a book. It is a real force and again should be utilised.

The positive thinking techniques we use all centre on outer activities that a person who wants to get well again can use to that end. *Meditation* is an inner activity which, also, subtly leads to an increase in the will to live. Interestingly, people who *meditate* learn acceptance, they can go with the flow and while their basic preference becomes very much pro-life they can accept what occurs during that lifetime.

Once a diagnosis of cancer has been made, the expectation that you *can* live, if you want to, must be based on knowledge and reinforced by experience. The knowledge is there. Around 30 per cent of all cancers are cured by conventional methods and I feel sure that patients can do a lot to improve their chances. My own case and many others attest to that. This knowledge prompts people to have a go, to take that first step. As the body responds and they feel improvement, their belief is reinforced. They take the next step.

The ongoing process of healing is readily gauged by stress levels.

Healing = Harmony = Relaxation

So, if there is no stress in your life, you feel relaxed and well – great! Keep doing just exactly what you are doing.

If stress is apparent, re-assess your situation. It is good to reflect; perhaps contemplate how you react to stress now as compared to when your disease developed, particularly if you recognise that psychological profile. Again, if your methods of coping have not changed, it is a warning signal. You need to do more.

Meditation may be enough. Through its effects you may be able to stabilise your whole situation.

You may feel you need to actively work on it as well. You may find it best to avoid obvious causes of stress to begin with. If this means time off from work, or a holiday in a new environment for a while, be prepared to get your priorities right. Your family may think they want you today, but no doubt they would like to have you tomorrow as well.

It can be very helpful to analyse the causes of your stress. Write them down, talk them over with a good 'listening post', contemplate them. Seek to understand what constitutes stress for you, what you get out of it and what you can do to treat it. Remember, most stress is fear based, so look for the causes of fear.

Stress can also be approached on a spiritual level. Having a direct perception of a spiritual reality leads to a basic level of well-being and acceptance that makes stress far less of a possibility. It is a reality, to seek and look forward to such a direct perception of Truth. The satisfaction that comes with it transforms people's lives.

The overall key to success lies in acceptance, being able to accept yourself as you are. It lies in recognising that you have a weakness that you try to overcome and strengths you try to put to good use. With acceptance, you can try one hundred per cent in any situation. You realise that you can do no more and that anything less would be inappropriate. You can then live one day at a time, confident that there will be a tomorrow.

Finally, a state of poise can be reached where just living one day at a time is all right.

Chapter eleven

DEATH AND DYING

An integral part of living

Dying is okay. There is nothing wrong with dying. We are all going to do it one day, so why not enjoy it? I am not trying to be outrageous, trendy or flippant. Why let fear rob you of what could be the peak experience of your life? In death lies the answers. You will know. Stripped of your lower nature, your trappings, you will know who you really are. You will know consciousness is continuous, that life is continuous, and that your reality is spiritual. Perhaps that's what makes it a little 'scary'!

Death for me is an exciting prospect. While I admit to a gut fear of the physical process of dying, and a reluctance to leave those near and dear, it fills me with anticipation. Death is the ultimate adventure wherein the answers lie.

I seek a good death. I would prefer to be free of pain and drugs, but mostly I hope for the gift of a conscious death. To die suddenly, as in an accident or in my sleep, would be to miss a golden opportunity. I imagine my death as a gentle transition to another level of consciousness. Death means slipping off an old well-worn raincoat after a hard day's work, leaving the body and entering the warmth and security of a glowing home.

I love life. Life is great. And death is okay. I would rather death was much later. I have so much to do, give and learn. I am very much pro-life. But death is okay. It is part of life, too.

This book is about living, so it is about dying, too. Dying is a natural process. It is an integral part of life; we are all going to experience it this lifetime. So you do not need a terminal illness to prepare for death. In fact, the terminally ill often see their condition as a blessing as it does give them just that opportunity.

So often we become preoccupied with the mundane things of life and overlook what is happening inside. Who am I? Where am I going? What is life?

What if today was your last? Are you ready? *Are you?* Is your life's business complete? Have you used your life as you wanted? If this was your last day would you be doing anything different? If you were run over by a bus tomorrow would you die with a vulgar expletive on your lips, or could you produce an ineffable smile? The grace of a terminal illness lies in it providing the opportunity to focus on your *self*, to explore what is important for you and where your real priorities lie.

My preference has always been for life. I am still of the thought that a long life is of more value than a short one. I see plenty of short lives that seemed more valuable than long ones, but still I aim to help people live. Can you believe people who are open, free of fear, see death as just another part of living? People often express concern about whether a particular patient should concentrate on dying well, or still be aiming to recover. In my experience, patients always seem to have this built-in instinct that directs them to concentrate on techniques for helping them in living, or techniques for helping them in dying. Can you believe that when they are open, free of fear, those techniques are one and the same? They both aim for wholeness.

Our cancer support groups have a twelve-week cycle of discussions. When we began, people attended regularly until the 'Death and Dying' week. About one-third of our usual number turned up! Now, under rather forceful urgings, most come and when they do they find a surprise. Talking of death and dying leads to a release, a letting go which produces a significant change towards improving quality of life. Most problems with death are fear-based, and once knowledge dispels this fear and love is active in people's hearts, another great barrier to real self-realisation is removed.

So why has the fear of death been so prominent in so many lives and in cancer patients particularly? My youthful memories of death still revolve around a scene from the film *Pollyanna*. A black, vulturous minister climbs into a white pulpit for the Sunday oratory and glares at the fresh-faced, life-loving congregation. 'Death strikes unexpectedly', he bellows. The congregation cringes and shrinks under his verbal fear-based tirade. I remember little of the rest of the film as I hid for most of it under my seat.

It fascinates me to note that in Victorian times images of death had an air of ethereal peace with quite a note of triumphant heroism. Then sex was dirty and taboo, the thing not to speak of. Our society has changed. Today sex is analysed under the full light of day while death is shrouded in mystery and fear.

Perhaps that fear of death is understandable. It has its roots in our physical and psychological nature. A physical fear of death is a natural part of our self-preservation instinct. It's the thing that makes us jump back from cliff edges or out of the way of speeding buses. It is a protective mechanism of the body and personality, of the lower self. It produces that gut fear that is quite acceptable and natural.

The psychological fear is of three types:

- fear of leaving the known – the things that we enjoy on the physical, emotional and mental levels
- Fear of the process of dying
- Fear of entering the unknown

Again, knowledge dispels fear. We can work towards accepting our leaving of this world, understanding the process of dying, and having confidence in what lies beyond. To do so requires a fearless honesty with self and good communication with others. Relatives, friends and counsellors can all contribute, but it takes good timing to discuss this area with others. The patient should be the one to start such a sharing. Helpers can give prior indications that they are willing to talk of death. As not all people are comfortable enough with it themselves to talk openly of it with others. But it is not the sort of subject area wherein you can waltz up to someone with a major illness and say, 'Well, let's talk about death and dying today'. You must wait until they are ready.

However, I strongly recommend to both patient and helper that they do make the effort to talk about it. Expressing oneself and sharing one's thoughts and feelings with another gives a tremendous sense of release, in this area perhaps more than any. It is remarkable to see the fears 'letting go' when a true heart-to-heart exchange takes place.

At one session Joan, the mother of a young cancer patient, broke down when we discussed death and dying. It was as if a release valve had been opened. All her pent-up emotions and fears flowed out. A wonderful thing happened. All the cancer patients there felt such compassion for her that they all reassured her. It was okay. It was good for her to express her emotions, her fear. To start with, most of them envied her being able to do so. They all said in different ways that death was all right if that was what happened. But her young child was not going to die. In fact, he has made remarkable progress against the odds. But that session and her catalytic effect transformed the other patients. It was as if a cloud of anxiety was lifted from them as they spoke openly and earnestly of their fears and attitudes on death. Not only did they convince her, they convinced themselves, that death was okay. I am sure the boost in the level of well-being of the group was physically noticeable after that session.

There are many things to talk of with death and dying. You may find these different sections useful catalysts to get a conversation going at home.

Children's attitudes

Children begin with a wonderful, inherent simplicity. They are then very much influenced by the attitudes and actions of those around them. Children, when they first become aware of death, accept it as part of the natural proceedings. Up until the age of three, death is no different from any other separation. Auntie Flo may be on a holiday or she may be dead – she's not here at the moment but she will probably be back later. Little children live in the now.

Around the age of three an awareness of death as being different to other separations begins to dawn. I well remember when Rosemary, aged three, first realised something had 'died'. We had been looking after a baby ring-tail possum for the previous ten days. It had been very ill to start with. Because it was so small, Grace and I, and sometimes Rosemary, had been carrying it in a little fur-lined bag against our bodies to keep it warm. We slept with it, too and this morning we woke to find it had died during the night. Rosemary bounced in to us as usual and asked to hold the possum. We had had no time to 'plan' our approach so Grace said, 'It's down the back'. Rosemary went down and took it from its bag. Holding the little creature in her hand she looked across to me and said, 'It's dead'. It was one of those delightful moments. She was looking to me to see how she should react, and I was looking to her to see how I should react. We both just looked at each other for quite sometime, me trying not to put any loadings on her wondering what to do. Rosemary looked back at the possum. 'It's eyes are open'. Another quick look towards me, and, 'We ought to bury it'. So out we went and installed the little animal under a rose bush, had a moment's silence and back in for breakfast. Back to full and exuberant life, and the possum was only ever mentioned in casual, open terms if the conversation passed his way.

Children at this age have a wonderful sense of the cyclic nature of life. They instinctively know that plants grow from seeds, mature, flower, produce more seeds and die. They fully expect those seeds to grow and bloom again next season. They feel the same way about animals and people, too. They accept that they have gone for a while, but they will be back.

When the fox killed Rosemary's pet goose, Cheepey, I am sure Grace and I were more upset than she was. They had a beautiful relationship. Rosemary had found Cheepey half-stuck in his egg kicked out of the nest by his mother. She took over and raised him to be a beautiful, placid, friendly bird.

We saw the fox, whom we half affectionately knew as Freddy, in the act of taking him, and so recovered the body. Well I remember Rosemary trudging up the orchard with Cheepey's large bulk clasped to her body, his long neck dangling at her side. It was heart-rending for me, a moment of great sadness. I felt great anger towards the fox and great compassion for Rosemary. Rosemary had not cried or appeared upset after the first moment of realising who it was that the fox had taken. 'Is it Cheepey, Daddy?' she had asked in a small faltering voice. 'Yes, it's Cheepey, Rosemary.' 'Rotten Freddy!' was her exasperated reply.

We buried Cheepey under a wisteria. Rosemary talked a lot of him in the weeks to come. 'Remember when I used to do this with Cheepey?' and 'Remember when Cheepey did this?' were common phrases for some time. Quite spontaneously Rosemary also said, 'When the goose eggs hatch next year, Cheepey will be among them and I will have him as a pet again'. She was quite happy to wait for the seasons to go around.

This cyclic approach is very similar to that Eastern philosophy of reincarnation and one I feel comfortable with. Children have a natural appreciation of this.

Often at this early age, however, they will also associate death with physical damage. This is because most often they become aware of it by finding a dead bird or having the family dog squashed on the road. The fear of death being associated with mutilation can be very real.

We need to be very careful with little children so as not to reinforce that fear. How often do parents find children with a dead animal or bird and snatch it away saying, 'You don't want to look at that'. Rubbish. The parent may not want to look at it, but the child is magnetically drawn. They know that herein lies a great mystery, the mystery of life and death. If it is snatched from them by fearful parents they are left wondering, 'Why is it fearful? Why shouldn't I look at it?'

Similarly, it is most important to talk of death in the family situation. If a relative or friend dies, children are bound to be curious. Do not fob them off, even if it is painful for you to talk of it. Answer their questions as openly and honestly as you can. Expressing your grief is fine, too; grief is a natural part of death also. But try to keep fear out of it.

Try to talk in those terms to which the child can relate. I always laugh at the reply to a child's puzzled question, 'Where has my puppy gone?' 'Don't worry, dear, he's gone to a loving God.' The child looks up in disbelief and you can read his mind. 'A loving God? But my puppy is gone! No *loving* God would take my puppy away!'

Choose your words carefully and try to make sense. If you do not fully understand, it is better to share your own thoughts and feelings, even if they include confusion, than to attempt to gloss over them with a platitude.

Frequently, by the age of five, the child is beginning to think death has a character all of its own. While they still accept its cyclic nature, they feel as if death is like a bogeyman who comes and steals things away in the night. This continues on until the age of around nine years when the realisation sets in that death is the permanent end of that particular biological life form. Responses then are very much tempered by previous experiences, cultural backgrounds and circumstances. In other words, they react like adults who can display any of the full range of emotions – from peaceful silence to outbursts of rage.

Responses to death can be very complex. Often they are loaded with guilt. A child might have told his brother, 'Why don't you go and drop dead!' or 'Do that again and I will kill you'. If brother does get run over by a bus the child may feel involved in actually causing it. Often adults feel guilty. 'If only I had done more for her'. 'If only . . .'.

Not infrequently it is anger that is felt. 'How could they go and leave me in this predicament?' 'Why has Daddy left me?'

Obviously these negative type emotions should preferably be worked through before someone dies. Again, a terminal illness can be a blessing here, as people do have the opportunity to put their affairs in order, including their relationships. Jenny, who has been managing her very difficult physical condition for far longer than she was expected to survive, has worked well with her family in this regard. They all want her to recover, as she does too, but they have talked of the possibility of her dying. Her teenage daughter eventually confided that she was worried that her mother would not be there when she reached those crucial times in her life like leaving home and getting married. Her mother prepared tapes for her and collected a dowry together. She hopes her daughter will not need a recorder, that she will be there to meet the needs in person, but she is content to know that the situation is covered.

Discussing dying

It is so important, for couples particularly, to talk of their feelings and attitudes. What would you do if the other died? A friend had a wonderful, loving, truly harmonious relationship with his wife. After she died, however, he was quite distraught because he did not know what his wife would want him to do with their three children and all the eventualities that arose. Now, I am sure those two thought as one. They discussed the whole spectrum of life together, but not death. So he was left wondering and went through a great deal of anguish trying to make those decisions that should have been straightforward.

Consider these things. Do make the effort to talk of them. Don't avoid the hard questions like the issue of remarriage. Do give expression to any preferences you have for funeral arrangements, cremation or burial, and the like. If someone in a terminal situation starts to talk of death or dying, don't try to change the subject. If old Granny starts telling you what she wants to leave to you, don't patronisingly pass her off as being morbid with, 'Now, now, you don't want to talk like that'. She does. It is very important for people to be able to express themselves in this area, and unless they have the opportunity of a sympathetic ear, a lot may go unresolved. Do get your will in order. This is not morbid, but practical and considerate.

Stages of dying

So what of the process of dying itself? Elisabeth Kubler-Ross has done more to acquaint the public with this than anyone else. Working with the dying and being sensitive to their needs rather than her own, she identified five now classic stages that dying people pass through. These are explained in her book on *Death and Dying*.[18] In my experience, it needs to be stressed that these stages overlap considerably and people can travel back and forth between them. I also see a secondary pattern emerging. But it is very useful to be aware of these stages.

1   Denial
'It's all a mistake. The X-rays were mixed up in the lab'. I remember thinking this one myself – for about two seconds, and then I accepted it was for real. Some people cannot, and go from place to place seeking a new opinion. Others just refuse to believe that they have a potentially life-threatening illness.

2   Anger
'Why me?' 'Why did I get it, why not old George down the road?' Again, some people take this emotion to its extreme and go through a particularly difficult time.

3   Bargaining
'If I go back to Church regularly, then perhaps I will live another six months'. The thing about bargaining is that it involves a fantasy. You may well go to Church, find ingredients missing in your life, make changes and recover completely. No sense of bargaining

there – just take appropriate action. Any self-help techniques could be bargaining unless the motivation was right.

Bargaining techniques are not sustained. Because they are based on fantasy they do not get carried through. Genuine self-help techniques are sustainable because they bring results, even if those results do not change the physical situation. It is important, with cancer particularly, not to view it as a game of winners and losers with death the end-point. Cancer is an intensification of the game of life. It is a game of winners and losers, but success is marked by wholeness, peace and harmony. Death may still be involved. This is not a cop-out or rationale to justify death. Some people live lives of little quality, others live dying with dignity, poise and accomplishment. I think particularly of Robert, a senior Government man who came to us with advanced secondary myeloma. He was depressed and feeling terminal. He rapidly became enthused about *meditation*, a thing he had actively resisted until this point. He changed his diet, and his attitudes. He received great support from his wife and they spent an exciting, growing and happy six months. A brain tumour then asserted itself and he died quickly. His wife told me that those last six months were the most meaningful of their time together. Was that period of six months enough? She stressed she felt no sense of having 'lost' in the situation.

So I see people who accept their situation and work with it. Incredibly they often feel that death is of far lesser importance than what they are gaining through the process. For most in our groups this third stage, then, is one of *taking appropriate action* and it leads on to *acceptance*. This is a sustainable acceptance that carries them through getting well or through dying. They can accept life.

4 Depression

'I don't want to know anyone.' Patients can go through periods of deep depression where everything is 'wrong'. They are then very difficult to help and very insular. I feel this happens when they are beset by the physical reality of their situation and preoccupied with thoughts and fears of their lack of immortality. Often, however, this can be interspersed with moments of great clarity when their spiritual realities appear more real and comforting.

5 Acceptance

'It's okay to die.' Patients may be insular or not, but are characterised as being at peace. Nearly everyone, it seems, unless they are absolutely overwhelmed by fear or anger, passes through this stage before dying. Physical pain often melts away and there is a great sense of calm. For people who work at it, this stage can be a wonderful peak experience. If shared, it can offer families and friends an experience they are unlikely to get in any other way.

It is as well to realise that friends and relatives can also be involved in this five-stage process. A little of them is dying, too, as they lose someone near and dear. They, too, can need help to get it right before a death. People who exhibit love and faith have death marked by kindness and compassion. People who express competition and fear often find confusion and loneliness. The art of dying lies in the art of living.

Grief

While I am sure it is possible to accept death as a transition and a positive event, most people in our society feel that grief is the appropriate emotion. There is no doubt that the physical loss of someone you love is something you would prefer to avoid. I think of my old Granny, however. She was a wonderful lady. She lived a long, healthy life giving great service and joy to those around her. We travelled in Europe with her in her eightieth year and she gave us a new, fresh perspective as we battled to keep up with her unflagging energy. When she died she had completed a really valuable life. I felt as close to her as anyone. I felt at her funeral we should have been thankful, even joyous, for that wonderful spirit and life. Grief just did not seem an appropriate emotion. She had lived a full life and was going on to new experiences.

Perhaps this attitude is easier to adopt with an elderly relative where the relationship is loving and uncluttered. It is more difficult when children are involved or a lot of business is left undone. So, again, get it right before they die. Work on 'living right' and you automatically work on 'dying right'.

However, there are some useful aids for helping someone who is grieving. Most of us would find it difficult to help another through a period of grief. It is always an emotionally charged time. What should we say, or do? Faced with indecision it would be easy to do nothing, but by using some simple principles we can be very helpful indeed. The aim is to communicate, to give the grieving person the opportunity to express their thoughts, and particularly their feelings, and for you to communicate your care and empathy.

So do not try to change the subject. Do not make light of it, but share in the difficulties it can produce. By being prepared to talk of the person who has died and the situation they face through the loss of that person, you give them the opportunity to express themselves. Often only emotions and feelings will come out and logic may not be a part of them.

Quite often negative emotions may come out. Guilt, anger, despair, even rage, are just as likely to appear as gratitude, acceptance and love. Do not develop an argument by trying to counter negative feelings with positive ones. What is being expressed is an emotional response and if it is not released in the early days after the death, it will remain. Repression of such emotions and feelings may cause bitterness and disillusionment. Frequently this means that your role is to say very little. It is certainly harder to be a listener than a talker and often the grieving person will say the same thing over and over. They are expressing feelings, not logic. Given the opportunity to do this they will then be cleared and at the next meeting a more logical discussion of the situation will be possible. Sometimes the initial talks will lead to tears, so have the courage to let this happen if it is needed because it allows the person to 'let go' that inner tension which, in turn, leads to release.

Action reinforces your own feelings, so find something to actually do for the grieving person. Whether it be taking around a prepared meal or accompanying them on a day's outing, the physical act shows you really do care. Remember that at the time of a funeral there is always a lot to do and a great deal of support comes forward. Four to six weeks later, however, everyone is getting back to their own immediate concerns and it is at this later stage that the loss will be most noticed by those closely affected. Make a note on your calendar to call on them, and to help your friend to find new interests and directions. Helping them to do things for themselves is a start, but once they are helping others life is well under way again.

Possibly the most exciting aspect of dying is the work that has been done on the near-death experience. Raymond Moody in *Life after Life* talks of his experiences with people who have been revived after being clinically dead.[19] Their experiences are remarkably similar. They were struck by their feelings of calmness and lack of fear. Even people who were involved in severe accidents and suffered serious physical injuries were aware at the time of the accident that they felt no pain. They felt like a calm observer – yes, an observer, standing to one side or, more commonly, looking down on the scene surrounding their physical body. People who have been on operating tables and lapsed into clinical death have often been able to recall the words spoken by the doctors and what was done to revive them. One of our group who experienced this recalled her doctor saying, 'Don't give up on me now, you bitch – breathe!' It was a red-faced doctor who verified using those words.

Many have then experienced a sensation of leaving the vicinity of their body and passing down what seems to be a tunnel. It is often a tunnel of light, or there is a light at the end of this tunnel. Again, the feeling is one of comfort and security, no fear. Frequently there is someone known and loved by the patient at the other end as if to greet them. This experience is not recalled by people with a yen for spiritualism, but ordinary everyday people. A recent study showed that 40 per cent of all people who have been clinically dead, recounted some or all of these experiences. It is then as if they reach a threshold – to pass over it would be irreversible and death would occur. Obviously, people telling these stories came back, and usually they felt a compelling reason to do so. They either had unfinished business or a sense of mission. So one of our group, a devout Catholic, got to the end of her tunnel to be met by her deceased grandfather. 'You're too early, lass. You have to go back, for the children.' She recovered from surgery and now has a profound knowing that death is okay.

This is the exciting thing. People who have this near-death experience are left with a feeling of comfort and peace. Death is nothing to fear. In fact, it is described as a very pleasant process.

I had a similar experience following my amputation. I had an adverse drug reaction and felt as if my awareness was becoming out of time with my body. Feeling strange, it was as if I was watching myself call for a nurse and as if I was watching someone else trying to explain what was happening. Then I lost awareness of my surrounds. I recorded in my diary that I felt as if I was being propelled along a hose in a stream of water. If you have ever pointed a stream of water to the sky on a sunny day and seen the stream break into beads of sparkling light, you will know how I felt. It was as if I reached the end of the hose and had a glimpse of a glorious array of cascading beads of light. I felt strongly that if I kept going with those beads I would not return. It was a beautiful sight. I took one glimpse and said to myself, 'No thanks, not yet'. Soon my awareness returned to the hospital room.

At the time I wondered if I had hallucinated, or had experienced something more. It had been so real at the time, however, that I felt sure I had been through a genuine experience. It left me knowing that death was okay. It is all very well to rationalise and talk about it, but, after an experience like that, you *know*.

This positive view of death is backed by a philosophy that sees death as an integral part of life. *Meditation* has enhanced that feeling by adding to my appreciation of spiritual reality. So I would like to think that just as I can celebrate all the other life events, birth, marriage, childbearing, maturity, so I should be able to celebrate death. While I accept that remorse, anguish and grief are real and need to be dealt with, I look to give thanks for life and wish people well in their new phase of it, after death. I try not to cling to old memories and so bind people who have new directions to explore. I seek to avoid complications by communicating well with people before they die, seeking to explore the practical issues as well as feelings, thoughts and attitudes.

An approach to death

It is well to have the courage to develop a concept of what you think will happen when you die. You might like to meditate and contemplate it. This is not a ghoulish thing, but a useful prerequisite for approaching death in an open way. Again, you do not need a life-threatening illness to gain enormously from this. You will probably find fears well up and it is good to analyse them and use the techniques to let them go. Letting go of attachments is the key.

It is also good to discuss the practical details of what life might be like if you were to die. What schools should the children attend? Should outside help come into the family? And so on.

Whatever else you do, do talk about this vital area. It is probably the hardest conversation to get started, but everyone is amazed at how well it flows once it begins. Such sharings lead to increased bonding between families and friends, heighten peace of mind and do a great deal to enhance quality of life.

Perhaps the most beautiful comment came from four-and-a-half-year-old Anna. When asked by her mother what she thought had happened when her grandmother died, Anna paused to reflect for a moment, then replied, 'Well, Mummy, just the *living part* went out of her.'

Chapter twelve

THE PRINCIPLES OF HEALING

Health in the balance

Healing is another integral part of the process of life itself. In seeking to understand the healing process we can compare it to a journey between two great cities – one called Disease, the other Health. Disease is known by suffering, separation and restriction, Health by joy, wholeness and freedom. The journey between the two is that of Healing.

It would be tempting to say the journey was on a purely physical level and that being free of physical symptoms assured a place in the city of Health. Experience tells us otherwise. We see people of sound body beset by mental anxiety. We see people of no purpose wandering the byways with no direction. We see others wracked by physical disease whose inner light shines strong and pure. So this is a metaphorical journey indeed. A journey of personal evolution.

The paths between any great cities are many and varied; the routes people take between Disease and Health are diverse indeed. It is as if we are born somewhere along that route with our own particular inborn level of health and our own range of talents with which to work. As we grow, we respond to the environment around us. Some of us, then, pass our days being merely bumped along by the external events of life. In what appears to be a waste of a grand opportunity, these make little progress as their life passes by. Others do move off in search of a better clime, but find no compass to guide them. Often they stumble deep into the city of Disease before realising they are on the wrong track. Then comes the test, to change direction, to learn to read the map and head back to the security of Health.

Those brave ones who do dare to tread the path to Health,

unprovoked by such a stay in the compelling city of Disease, are the ones in life I admire most. Those who value life and its opportunities, who respect their deeper nature, and their body and work to better it, have really grasped the purpose of their life. They are the ones who, when you meet them along the path, exude the joy of the search and uplift all they encounter.

The paths between the two cities are as varied as the travellers. There are narrow, winding lanes for those who wish to dally; there are wide, direct highways for those with purpose and perseverance. And for some, although few it seems, there are the airports where, spreading wings, it is possible to fly direct to the destination. All along these routes are towns and places of interest. Some are unrewarding, mere dalliances and distractions along the way, while other stops add quality and enrichment.

As the travellers move along the separate routes, their paths often cross. When they do, it appears to the passing individuals that they are heading in opposite directions. Without the benefit of a grander map they might be tempted to say the other was wrong in pursuing such a course, exclaiming: 'Follow me. My way is the best, the only path to Health'. Those with a grander sense of vision, however, acknowledge their fellow seekers and bless them as they move on their way, for direction comes with discovering that this is more than a physical quest. Disease: dis-ease. The word says it all – lack of ease, lack of balance, lack of harmony. Health is harmony and the purpose of life is to seek harmony on all levels of our being – physical, emotional, mental and spiritual.

The further we journey, the more we realise we are responsible for our own position on the map of life, and that we must accept that responsibility. We see that life has a pattern and we are an integral part of it. We are intimately involved with the complex pattern of events that has resulted in our being in our current situation. Maturity comes with finding our position on the map and accepting that position. Then, if we are strong enough not to indulge in looking back with guilt or regret, we can chart our own course and take the first steps towards Health.

Some of us find it is hard to accept responsibility for being in our present position. Particularly if physical disease is evident, it is far easier to blame something or someone else for our own misfortune and so feel a victim of circumstances. But some time, somewhere, the realisation dawns and we appreciate that the pattern of the life we have been leading has determined our current circumstances. We are responsible, just as we can be in control.

If our past pattern has produced the symptoms of disease, and now we are seeking to re-establish health, we must be brave enough to look for a change in direction. Change is required to establish the pattern that leads to Health. Some can make that change almost instantaneously. With the speed of jet travel they can relocate themselves in new and happy surrounds. For most, however, the journey becomes a process, *the healing process*. It develops as a series of changes that gradually lead to the place of their dreams. Commonly, the first steps are superficial ones and there is a preoccupation with the obvious physical steps that are needed to be taken. So patients journey to places of physical treatment, change their diet, begin to exercise. These outer things are easy to start with, easy to work on. As they come under control, the effort becomes more profound. The inner work begins. The need to change fundamental attitudes and direction becomes apparent. To change just one really basic trait for the better is a major challenge for any lifetime.

So, where is the map? Where is the compass? What can guide us through this maze? In essence it really is very simple. Once our basic course is realigned with harmony, once harmony is the prime motivation, then healing is under way. The more harmony in our actions, attitudes and spirit, the better our quality of life and the closer we move towards that wonderful city of Health.

Harmony comes with peace of mind, so as we seek peace of mind, we seek Health. If, at every step along the way, peace of mind is the basic criterion that must be satisfied, then each and every step would be a good one, one that takes us in the right direction. To begin with, the physical may lag behind, but in terms of inner development, once harmony is the aim and peace of mind the governing principle, then progress is surely under way.

In fact, once we are free of physical symptoms we often discover that the journey has only just begun. While many find that healing their physical ailments does bring great personal spiritual growth, they soon realise that the true aim of the process of healing is really synonymous with the aim of the process of life itself – to seek harmony on all levels. Their spirit leads the way and often aspires to journey beyond the place where their physical and psychological reality dwells and works.

So often the journey produces tension, a tension of growth, as the spirit leads the personality towards its goal. If this tension is creative, the path runs smoothly. If the personality lags or resists, then bumps abound. When the prime motivation is peace of mind, the journey to Health is steady indeed.

The means to Health, the paths of healing, run on many levels and are extremely varied. To clarify the map a little we can summarise some of these many and varied routes.

Aids to healing

Physical

1 Medical

All these areas require specialised advice. This is merely an introductory overview of some of the possibilities. If you feel drawn to a particular area, then seek help from the appropriate qualified practitioner.

Surgery: In statistical terms, surgery does little to extend the overall life expectancy for most cancer patients. However, it can be useful in individual cases such as melanoma. It can also be helpful by removing existing tumours and so take a load off the body, giving it time and a better opportunity to prevent recurrences. It is best used when tumours can be removed en masse, with nothing left behind.

Chemotherapy: The side-effects need to be weighed against the benefits. In some situations it is very effective, but quality of life can suffer and needs to be watched.

Radiation: This is often used to reduce pain and can do so, particularly when bone is involved. It is effective as a treatment in a limited number of situations but, personally, is my least favoured form of treatment.

Immunotherapy: This is an experimental area in conventional medicine. For example, BCG vaccination, which aims to stimulate the immune system, can be helpful in some cases.

Hormonal therapy: Some tumours can be hormone responsive, for example some breast cancers and prostate cancers.

2   *Paramedical*
Nutrition : See Chapters 7 and 8.

Exercise : See Chapter 5.

Massage : See Chapter 10. Foot massage is good – see books on Reflexology and/or the Metamorphic Technique.

3   *Natural therapies* (There are two mainstreams):
(i)   Chinese Medicine: This is best approached through a trained Chinese doctor or someone well versed in this total approach. It considers body, mind, and spirit, and is run through with a deep philosophy. It utilises herbs, massage, counselling, acupuncture. I find it fascinating and would like to study it more deeply. I use acupuncture in my veterinary practice. However, I wonder if, in its entirety, it is not better suited to the Chinese themselves than to those of Western traditions. Certainly it has a great deal to offer.

(ii)   Naturopathy: This is probably best approached via a good iridologist. Iridology is the science of relating changes in the iris to changes in the body. In competent hands it is a valuable diagnostic aid and a wonderful aid to prevention. Through it, weaknesses in the body can be detected before they produce physical symptoms. A good naturopath would then strengthen these weaknesses by drawing on nutrition, lifestyle advice, herbs, manipulation, massage, homeopathy, etc. These can all amount to a useful way of maximising your potentials. It is a good avenue for building up your natural defences.

Psychological

Positive thinking: See Chapter 5, including the healing environment factors.

Stress management: See Chapter 10.

Affirmation: See Chapter 5.

Visualisations: See Chapter 5.

Meditation: See Chapters 2 and 3.

Spiritual

Healing relies on rediscovery and direct perception of your own spiritual reality or belief system. See Chapter 13.

Psychic Healing

There is a need to share some of the experiences which Grace and I had with paranormal healing phenomena, notably psychic surgery in the Philippines. Firstly, it is widely known that I have benefited from such treatment and I am sure this needs clarifying. Secondly, such psychic phenomena are most intriguing. If they can be shown to be genuine in just one instance, the implications are vast indeed. I find it a fascinating area.

Warning: If, however, this field of endeavour or this type of conjecture is not to your taste, please do not be put off by it. We have had remarkable experiences and seek to explain them. If I do not do so adequately, that is *my* shortcoming. The other more concrete things covered in the book to this point stand in their own right, and in our experience are fully justifiable. What follows is the product of experience, reading, conjecture and contemplation. It may shed some light on what is to us a truly wonderful area – the mysterious area of healing.

It is interesting to note how many types of paranormal phenomena are cropping up today, and the interest they are producing. Debate on psychic surgery has been intense for quite a few years. Reports of miraculous cures have been countered with claims of quackery, sleight of hand and the use of chicken's blood and tissues of non-human origin. Uri Geller has bent spoons and started clocks. At the same time, the Russians experiment with psychokinesis, that is, moving objects without touching them, using psychic energy alone. If these things are talked of openly, what experiments are going on in secret?

In the healing arena Kirlian photography is being used to distinguish between healthy and diseased tissues. A sophisticated technique of photography, it reveals what is claimed to be the health aura. Clairvoyant healers now, and in ages gone by, have reported this subtle energy emanating from their patients. Acupuncture has already been accepted into the conventional treatment repertoire despite there being no conventionally accepted explanation for its means of action.

We are getting a lot of hints, demonstrations of the possibilities. Frequently, patients in dire need are being drawn by such phenomena, often turning their backs on conventional treatments. Patients can see that there are practical benefits to be gained. But there is a great need for balance – the ability to decide what treatment and when. Likewise, many treatments have a synergistic or complementary effect. Consideration of diet, meditation, and positive thinking, should be essential in the treatment of cancer. While many are choosing to rely on these methods alone, I feel they also act to potentiate any other form of treatment, whether orthodox or not.

My own healing has been similar to putting the pieces of a jigsaw puzzle together. After the initial surgery, diet and meditation were complemented by acupuncture, iridology, psychic surgery, massage, a short course of chemotherapy, radiesthesia, and on through twenty-seven different healing techniques. Of all these, the only thing I felt to have a negative effect *for me* was the radiation treatment. [We have included books that delve into each of these areas in References and Further Reading.]

It is interesting, however, that the people involved with each form of treatment were almost universally convinced that their treatment was all I needed to get well again. I was fortunate to be led from one to another by the way circumstances arose, and my training, helped me to judge what I needed to presevere with. Few of the individuals involved could see their treatment as *part* of a process or see any unifying thread running through them all.

This is the challenge: Was it a random exercise, a clutching at straws, or was there an underlying principle at work?

It is best not to get bogged down discussing the pros and cons of each of my treatments. All the medicos who have looked at my history agree that it goes outside normal expectations. There is no conventional medical explanation for why I should be here. But, as with all things, there is room for debate on details and I would prefer to consider the principles involved.

So far we have been doing just this. We have been considering the patient's role in cancer and what they can do to help themselves back to health. While the principles of diet, positive thinking and nutrition break enough new ground, the area of psychic surgery introduces us to a whole new frontier.

Chapter thirteen

THE MYSTERY OF HEALING

The message of the extraordinary

When my leg was amputated in 1975 there had been no other sign of the cancer. It reappeared, however, and *osteogenic sarcoma-secondary cancer* was diagnosed later that year. I was told that the medical options of chemotherapy and radiation were not likely to improve my chances of living more than another three to six months and that they would have unpleasant side-effects. I was also told that the cancers were likely to double in size every month.

Concentrating on meditation and diet, however, saw no growth at all over the first three months. Then through a combination of factors, mostly to do with my trying to do too much each day and so creating new stresses, I deteriorated rapidly. Initially the seering pain of sciatica running down my left side restricted my mobility. Then my weight fell away and I was confined to bed. Finally it was confirmed that my right kidney was obstructed and severely swollen. I had reached my lowest point.

In desperation Grace and I left for the Philippines in March of 1976. I weighed little over six stone [about thirty-eight kilograms] compared to my normal nine (twelve before my leg was amputated). My colour was likened to that of a jaundiced custard. Pain forced me to lie down except when it was absolutely necessary to move.

We were motivated by the conviction that I would still recover, but we knew little of what to expect. We had heard of the Filipino healers from several people, notably an aunt and friends who had helped to introduce me to the dietary regime some months earlier. They had given us the address of one healer, one young Filipino boy whom they thought might be helpful, and one hotel. While excited by the possibilities, and open to them, I was basically sceptical and certainly critical in my approach to the healers. The first thing we did in the Philippines was to buy a movie camera. If I was to be tricked, I wanted to record it.

Two days after arriving, I had my first operation performed by a small, shy, Filipino healer. Travelling to his house early in the morning, we were met by his cousin who doubled as business manager. He told me that after the treatment I was to return to my hotel and rest a few hours. For twenty-four hours I was not to bathe or drink coffee, alcohol, or carbonated drinks. He also took twenty-two dollars from us, the amount this healer charged in those days. It was the first and last time we were asked for money.

Most of the healers work on a donation-only system. Most are very simple people of peasant background, with a strong Roman Catholic influence. They are not used to handling large sums of money. They say they are using a God-given power and accept what goods or money their patients can offer in return. Some who charged large amounts became preoccupied with material things and found their healing powers had waned. However, these were the exceptions, not the rule.

After the formalities, I was ushered into the operating theatre. This was a small bare room with a large wooden table to one side. The healer stood at its centre, flanked by two assistants. At his feet were two buckets. One was used as a repository for the bits and pieces that were removed, the other contained already bloodied water and was used for washing hands between operations. There was no pretence of sterile technique. We later learned that the healers have been shown to be able to destroy disease-causing organisms by merely passing their hands over them.

This day, there was no preamble. I was asked to strip to my shorts, to lie, back down, on the table, and to pray as best I knew. Under the circumstances, it was easy! The healer moved forward and quickly entered my abdomen with his fingers. He held his hands together, with fingers outstretched and just overlapping a little. I felt a pop, as when you poke a finger through a stretched rubber balloon. Grace was called over for a better look. As he pulled his hands apart she could see the lining of my peritoneal cavity and the tumour inside my pelvis. He then continued by taking some fresh tissue, similar to loose connective tissue, from the area. Blood welled up from within the incision, while there did not seem to be any bleeding from the skin itself. He finished by withdrawing his fingers, leaving a small pool of blood on my skin. When this was wiped away there was no scar visible. The performance was repeated in several other places and then I was unceremoniously told to get dressed and to return the next day. It had all taken five minutes.

I was excitedly asking Grace what she had seen as we returned to our hotel where I reluctantly agreed to lie down for a short rest. I slept extremely heavily for the next three hours, and after lunch I had another unexpected reaction. All my joints began to ache, one after another. I felt nauseous and colicky and my head began to spin. As these symptoms became more severe, I began thinking my surgeon's gloomy predictions might prove correct after all.

The Filipino boy, who soon showed that he had wisdom far beyond his years, was familiar with the problem, however, and said it frequently occurred. He explained that the healers were able to mobilise the body's own defences. Once this process was set in motion, it frequently produced a classic healing reaction with an intensifying of some or all of the patient's symptoms. Chronic conditions are often brought to a head and after a short, acute episode, healing progresses.

After a very uncomfortable twelve hours and a good night's sleep, I did, in fact, feel a great deal better. Within two days I had flushed all my analgesics down the toilet. Pain relief is a common sequel to this type of treatment and I am sure this is due to both a physical and psychological benefit. The healers are very aware of the psychological impact of this visually dramatic procedure. They recognise that if a patient believes that the disease which they have is normally terminal, then it takes something quite out of the normal to change that belief system and replace it with positive healing thoughts. They happily admit that their healing relies on its psychological impact as well as its physical effects.

We stayed on for four weeks and visited five healers during our first trip. Some people seek help from just one healer; others, like me, go to more. There are no set rules and it is important for the patient to accept responsibility for their own decisions and be guided by their own thoughts and feelings. The effects must also be put into perspective.

I returned from the first trip a stone heavier in weight, with no pain and with good mobility. My surgeon was amazed by the improvement. While there was no decrease in the actual cancer, there was no doubt that my general condition had improved dramatically. He said that he could not understand it; there was no medical explanation to account for it.

We continued to *meditate* and develop our dietary programme and look at any other avenue that might help keep this healing process going. Soon our movie films were back and confirmed what we had seen with our own eyes. It appeared that I had been operated on without anaesthetic or instrument. I had felt no pain, although I had bled and tissue had been removed. No scar remained as a visible sign of the procedures, but above all else, I had improved. *Something* had happened.

If just once a healer's hand, even a finger, had gone through my skin under these conditions, then my view of reality, my knowledge of physics and how surgery was possible, was quite inadequate to explain it.

There are three choices anyone faces when considering this phenomenon:

• It is a trick to be discounted.

• It is a miracle to be merely marvelled at and thankful for.

• It is a genuine phenomenon which requires explanation.

The history of physics is marked by the development of new theories that were required to justify previously unexplained phenomena. Whether it be Archimedes' 'Eureka!' in his bath, or Einstein's Theory of Relativity, all of physics has been a product of man's attempts to explain the world as he sees and experiences it.

I feel sure that the current wave of interest in psychic phenomena is really prompting us to look again at the nature of the world around us. The real message of the Filipinos is to offer a psychic signpost to a new awareness. For, if it is genuine – as I have come to believe it is – then it forces us either to take the easy way out and dismiss it as a miracle, or be brave and reconsider the nature of matter.

Most of us accept matter as being solid and finite. We sit on a chair and it feels solid enough. It looks solid. We tap it and it reassures us further by sounding solid. No doubt it has a taste and smell to add to its claims to solidity. But, is it? What is it made of – really? For it is the evidence of our five senses that we are relying on to call the chair solid. These five senses of touch, sight, sound, taste and smell are very helpful for us in day-to-day situations, but they have quite a limited range when compared to our modern precision instruments. If the range of sight of our eyes was just a little wider, we would all have X-ray vision. Imagine the difference just that one small change would have. Our view of reality would be transformed!

So, if we want to understand the nature of matter, we go to modern physics with all its marvellous technology. As the physicists analyse matter they look more closely at it, probing it with the aid of microscope, electron microscope and mathematical theory.

Most of us would be familiar with one of the results – the atomic concept of matter. The atom is a model for the ultimate building block. These building blocks are combined like pieces of a child's inter-locking building game to form all the substances we know.

The atom is represented as having a central nucleus with electrons circling it in orbit, much like the planets as they orbit the sun. But if we enlarge an atom to a size to which we can relate, we see just how 'holey' matter really is. For, if we represent that central nucleus by a pea a quarter-inch across, then, on that scale, the nearest electron would be the same pea-size; it would be 175 metres away and it would be going at the incredible speed of 2,000 kilometres per hour! Can there be all that space in what we consider to be solid? It has been calculated that if all the space was taken out of the atoms which make up the human body, the resulting mass would be smaller in size than a pin's head!

And it does not even stop there, for now the physicists have probed the atom still further. First they thought the nucleus and electrons were made of smaller and even smaller particles themselves. But now they say something even more startling: There is nothing solid there at all! The atom is merely the product of concentrated energy. *Matter is energy.*

We all know Einstein's famous equation, $E=mc^2$. But we seem to fall short of grasping its implications. E stands for energy, m for mass, and c for the speed of light. The equation is saying that mass is a product of energy and light – as esoteric a statement as formulated by any ancient sage.

This, to me, is the most remarkable thing of all. The modern physicists are becoming the New Age philosophers. For, as they probe deeper into the nature of matter, they are forced to look at energy and so seek to understand it. For, if all matter is made of energy, what makes the difference? Why does one 'block' of energy come together to build a rock, another a tree, another me?

The brave few physicists in the vanguard, who once more are prepared to ask that most vital question, 'Why?' are forced to introduce another concept – that of consciousness. They say that consciousness produces energy which, in turn, is interpreted by our five senses as the thing we call matter.

What a concept! Consciousness produces energy which produces matter. Thought precedes form. It leaves me concluding that my physical form is the result of the sum total of my consciousness. I must presume, therefore, that I and all those around me are all essentially reflections of our overall consciousness. Further, given our highly ordered world, I must presume an all-pervading consciousness to provide the basic framework in which it all happens.

Most humans have a similar view of reality; the world, as each one knows it, is basically similar. We interpret and respond to a basic universal energy pattern. Within this matrix we radiate our own sphere of influence – project our own thoughts and energies and so adjust the picture. For those capable of generating novel thought and projecting it with power, the whole picture can change at will. Reality is limited by our ability to conceive its possibilities.

Can we then understand more of the true nature of man? How can we formulate a model which takes into account these ideas of matter being consciousness and which also accounts for the phenomenon of the familiar physical world?

Why does some vast, all-pervading consciousness create the energy patterns that combine to produce the things we call atoms, which in turn combine in varied ways to produce the many things we call matter? And what, then, sparks this matter to produce a living organism with consciousness in its own right? And given all that, why do we see so much disease? We are now getting to the basic questions to which healers and patients need to find answers as they attempt to formulate a basic ethic with which to approach disease and its treatment.

Presently, all forms of paranormal phenomena are coming under scrutiny in the West. Parapsychology is an emerging science wrestling with these questions, but as yet no unifying principles have been commonly accepted.

However, if we turn to Eastern thought and metaphysics, there is a recurring model which both makes sense of the phenomena and provides a framework in which to operate.

Most major civilisations have had a tradition of an esoteric science in their culture. Being esoteric, it was hidden from the mainstream of the people but used by those initiated into its secrets in a very practical way. Despite the diversity of cultures, there is a remarkable agreement on basic principles. Even more remarkably, these principles relate to the concepts now being put forward by the modern physicists.

In the esoteric lore of the Ancient Egyptians, Chinese and Greeks, the Indians of North America and the Incas of the South American continent, the Polynesian Kahunas and Filipino healers, the Vedic seers of India, the early Christians and, more recently, the mediaeval alchemists and mystics of Europe, we find this recurring vision of man. It is esoteric in nature but still used in that very practical way. All these people saw man's physical body as being the end result of a series of interrelated and interdependent subtle levels of consciousness.

Basically, they saw man as being the sum total of seven levels of consciousness. To each level is assigned the form of an energy body. Only the energy of the physical body is dense enough to register immediately with the five senses and hence with the direct perception of another person. The other energy bodies can only be deduced by inference or perceived directly by clairvoyant or extra-sensory perception. If we consider the emotional – or astral level as it is frequently called – then I might think you are happy because I can see you smile and hear you laugh, but this does not mean I am appreciating your emotions directly or accurately. You may be putting on a front. A clairvoyant, however, might be able to see your emotional body directly, say in terms of subtle colour emanations, and so have a better idea of how you really do feel.

Similarly, healers say they base their diagnosis on perception of the subtle energy of the health aura.

The seven levels of consciousness are given various names, and I have used the following:

Divine	*Spirit*
Spirit Mind	
Spiritual-Intuitional Mind	Higher Self or Soul
Higher Intuitional Mind	
Mental-Intellectual Mind	
Emotional-Astral	Lower Self or Personality
Physical-Etheric	

The levels of consciousness are represented on an ascending scale purely for convenience as, in actuality, each is interrelated with the other.

The different Kingdoms are also related in this scheme. They are said to be concentrated in different areas of consciousness. The Mineral Kingdom is right in the physical level. A rock is a very physical thing! The Vegetable Kingdom is primarily in the physical, but peaks into the emotional. Experiments with lie-detectors are now confirming this ancient esoteric view by registering the emotional reactions of plants. This is well explained in *The Secret Life of Plants* by Tompkins and Bird.[20]

The Animal Kingdom is strongly involved with the physical and emotional levels and also has activity in the mental sphere.

Next comes Man, who has the most exciting prospects. We human beings are active on the physical, emotional and mental levels, and for us there is the possibility of making direct contact with higher levels of consciousness. For man there is this exciting distinction between the Personality and the Soul.

It is the personality or lower self, with which we are most familiar — our physical form, our emotions and thoughts. It is the thing that other people tend to know us as, the way we project ourselves to the world at large. But we have a soul also, the higher self or inner core of our being. It is the more permanent, purer, less complicated part of us.

Most of us are aware of the nature of our lower self or personality and work on this level. Only in moments of contemplation or inspiration do we make contact with the higher self or soul. The gap from personality to soul is the eye of the needle spoken of in the Bible, and the mind acts as the fulcrum between physical and spiritual man. Intellect must be transmuted into intuition to bridge that gap.

Our life purpose is to make that leap. Our goal is to be freed of the limitations of personality, and soar free as spiritual beings.

Death plays its part in this process by providing new beginnings. At death it is said the physical drops off and our consciousness persists in the other states. Usually, our new functional body is our astral body, or it may be a higher body, depending on our stage of development. In this altered state of consciousness, we develop further, before reincarnating into a new physical body for the purpose of advancing towards the state of perfection intended for all Man.

Reincarnation is governed by the Law of Karma, which is basically the spiritual law of cause and effect. Just as physically for every action there is an equal and opposite reaction, so also spiritually, as you sow so you shall reap.

Hence good actions have their rewards and bad ones need to be compensated. The aim of the game is to progress beyond the law of Karma. Then, free of the bonds of past activity, actions can be performed for their intrinsic 'correctness', without any thought as to the benefits they might produce. This leads to a state of enlightenment and reunion with the Divine — the destiny of all.

This concept helps to explain the seeming disparities around us and provides an incentive towards ethical, moral conduct in all situations.

But back to healing. The etheric body is vital to our considerations. It is the counterpart of our physical body. It is composed of a very subtle energy which is visible to sensitive people such as clairvoyants, as the health aura. It is this vehicle through which the other levels of consciousness impinge on the physical. It is centred on seven chakras. A chakra is a Sanskrit word used to describe the concentrations of this subtle energy which are said to be located in seven different regions of the spine and head. Each chakra is a reflection of one level of consciousness and, in turn, relates most directly to one particular endocrine gland.

The chakras can be thought of as energy transformers in an electricity grid. They relay energy to a network of power lines, which are called meridians or nadis, and which radiate throughout the physical body. The meridians correlate with the nervous system which in turn regulates the secretions from the endocrine glands. The hormones, so released, travel throughout the body via the blood and are instrumental in maintaining the body in its natural state of balance; hence the link from consciousness to matter. From the realm of consciousness, energy streams forth to vitalise etheric energy in the individual chakras. This energy then passes via the meridians to influence the nervous system's regulation of the endocrine glands. The hormones that then flow, via the blood, are vital in maintaining the physical body.

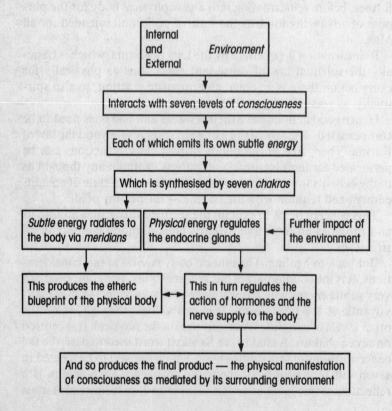

Internal and External *Environment*

↓

Interacts with seven levels of *consciousness*

↓

Each of which emits its own subtle *energy*

↓

Which is synthesised by seven *chakras*

↓

| *Subtle* energy radiates to the body via *meridians* | *Physical* energy regulates the endocrine glands | Further impact of the environment |

↓

| This produces the etheric blueprint of the physical body | This in turn regulates the action of hormones and the nerve supply to the body |

↓

And so produces the final product — the physical manifestation of consciousness as mediated by its surrounding environment

In this view, then, the physical body is the end result of formative energies as mediated by the etheric body which is in a state of dynamic flux. Its characteristics vary with the quality of the energies coming from the various formative levels of consciousness and with how its physical counterpart, the body, interacts with its own immediate physical environment.

Disease, then, can be due to purely physical causes, as in the rare case of a true accident, or, more commonly, is due to aberrations in the energy flows. Such aberrations reflect disharmony in the focal areas of the patient's attention. Many people now are focused primarily in the emotional sphere, while a growing number are centred in the mental. This fact is recognised by the growing attention being paid to psychosomatic diseases and the role of tension and anxiety in the production of disease.

Accepting our basically spiritual nature, it is easy to see the soul's overriding involvement and to consider disease in man as the end stage of disharmony between the soul and the personality — or friction between the higher self's attitudes and the lower self's actions. When such disharmony is left unresolved, it manifests as a physical reality so that we are forced to confront it.

Disease then provides an opportunity to progress beyond our limitations. To get the benefit of disease, to learn its real lessons, all aspects must be considered. Yet, in the immediate situation, it is often the physical condition which seems to be of prime importance. Most people living in the physical world do reject disease and death. They wish to continue here to experience and to progress as much as possible.

So just how do we set about healing a diseased body? If disharmony is the root cause, obviously anything that re-creates harmony will have a healing effect. If there is gross disease, however, the symptoms may be so severe and so physical, that it may not be possible for those involved to normalise the situation using only the energies available through esoteric avenues. There is no doubt this is a re-emerging science. While there are some people who can catalyse an immense change using these subtle energies, often it is necessary to alleviate the immediate situation with surgery and purely physical medicine, just to ensure a continuation of life.

This is a fine balance to strike. Physical treatments are tried and proven and will have a place for a long time, a fact often overlooked by over-zealous advocates of alternative medicine. But it is important to remember that it *is* physical medicine and frequently does not go beyond the treatment of the physical symptoms. Once the physical situation is stabilised, it becomes important to turn the attention to the underlying causes, and their correction, to effect a complete cure.

But before progressing here, I would like to reconsider the miracle of pure, physical surgery. Consider again the incredible trauma following a broken leg. It is easy to imagine the soft tissue damage, fragmented bones, and then perhaps a steel pin inserted to hold things in place. Yet, after medical intervention and the passage of a relatively short period of time, functions will return to normal and later X-rays will show little, if any, evidence of the damage. Just how can this be? What does initiate this truly wondrous healing which produces such magical effects?

We know quite a lot of the process, but what of the cause? We know a lot about how it happens. But why does it happen? I contend that a basic, relatively permanent blueprint of the body's form, as provided by the etheric body concept, does make sense of the situation. Although the physical form is traumatically altered in such accidents, the basic pattern, the etheric blueprint, remains. So, given the right conditions, healing will proceed and normal functions will return. It is a mistake to think that an outsider heals anything. A healer can be a most useful catalyst in the healing process, but the healer's true role is to create the correct conditions wherein the patient's *healing processes* themselves can re-create the normal state.

Consideration of this subtle energy model also accommodates the many other forms healing can take. Dietary considerations, for instance, act firstly on the physical level to purify the physical organism. But, as food has its own etheric energy, it can be a source of vitalisation on this level also. This is one reason why many people advocate the use of pure foods raised in as natural a way as possible. The more natural, the fresher and more vital our food, the more of this energy it has. Also it is believed that the subtle energy of food can be increased by being produced by a sensitive person, attuned to such ideas. On the other hand, the etheric value of much of the present-day mass-produced processed food must approach zero, or even have very negative connotations.

Meditation acts to balance the higher and lower selves. In a state wherein the physical, emotional and mental levels are removed from one's direct awareness, the intrinsic purity of the higher self can operate to reharmonise the etheric blueprint and so lead on to the recreation of the normal physical situation. Ainslie Meares says that *meditation* causes a return to a state wherein the immune system is induced to function normally. This causes the body to recognise and reject the presence of cancerous cells. This, he says, is mediated via an influence on cortisone levels. You can see the similarities in concept, the explanations being, to me, a matter of degree.

The Philippine healers are able to channel large amounts of direct healing energy. Sometimes they operate on a purely physical level. More often, however, they are operating on the precursive levels, notably the etheric and astral. Some are effective on the mental level, and a rare few heal on the spiritual level. Christ was a Divine Healer — capable of healing on any level.

This etheric energy of which we have been speaking has its global and universal counterpart, tied up with the all-pervading consciousness. It is on this energy that the psychic surgeons and other Faith healers draw. Most often merely accept it as God's gift of the Holy Spirit in action, and leave it at that. It is not too hard, however, to use our model and see that in effect they draw on the universal energy, focus it with their minds as a lens focuses the rays of the sun, and then emit it through their fingers in a beam of energy that can be compared to a laser beam.

This beam of energy can then neutralise the positive and negative charges holding tissues together at the molecular level. In the absence of these forces, the tissues separate and can be entered. When the energy is withdrawn the body's etheric forces reassert their blueprint effect so that the physical structures resume their normal state, with no scarring.

Alternatively, some people think that psychic surgery is performed through the action of harmonics. They believe that the healers are able to cause their hands to resonate in harmony with the tissue of their patients, so that the two can intersperse, much as two gases can intersperse.

Regardless of how it is achieved, once the healers are inside the body they utilise a magnetic facility which enables them to draw together the diseased energies and remove them. It is important to realise that frequently a change in phase does occur. That is, just as steam can be condensed to water, the healers seem able to concentrate the subtle formative energies associated with a physical symptom of disease and actually precipitate them into physical form. This is a demonstration of energy giving rise to matter – a true materialisation.

In the Philippines I was told that my bone tumours were too dense to be removed physically, but that the etheric energies associated with them could be taken away. My physical form would then return to match this normalised blueprint if I did not re-create the destructive etheric energies. So, after the initial boost, it became important to seek out the causes of disharmony within myself.

After the Philippines I had experienced a remarkable and generalised healing boost. Yet the tumours kept growing, although slowly. It was obvious to me I had not made the necessary changes in myself. Only after many more efforts, culminating in meeting Sai Baba, a Holy Man of India, was I really able to get free of my cancer problems.

There still remains the ongoing process which faces each one of us, that of developing a system in which to maximise our potentials, correct our shortcomings, and live in accord with our principles.

These energies can be channelled and used in a positive practical manner. [See Chapter 5 and Further Reading. The books listed allude to the possibilities.]

All of us do radiate these subtle energies. They are coloured by the quality of the channel through which they pass. It is vital, then, that we all seek to be as free as possible from complications within our own personalities.

Chapter fourteen

THE MYSTERY OF LIFE

A framework to live within

In this quest for a cohesive framework which accounts for the phenomenon of life as we know it, we must seek further still. What can we know of the mystery of Life?

We must look past the material world, past knowledge of the psyche and speculation of the psychic, to dwell on what lies at the core of life itself.

As modern man explores the world of the senses, many mysteries of the physical realities around us unfold, and our knowledge of things finite expands. But what of the infinite?

Most people who have explored the sensory world are firstly drawn by its comforts and pleasures. Our modern world is hallmarked by convenience and instant gratification. But, it seems, the more that people delve into the realms of physical delights, the more they feel something to be lacking, the more they seek a deeper sense of happiness. It would seem that modern society with all its marvellous technology, is reaching towards the outer limits of what is possible in the physical world. The problems that face us now can generally be solved on a physical level, but they remain as moral dilemmas.

Whether it be nuclear energy, test-tube babies, or organ transplants, the practical, physical know-how is generally there. But has wisdom kept pace with science? The problems that remain, the questions still to be answered, are now ethical, human considerations.

It takes but a moment's reflection to know that this is true. If, late at night, you go to bed, turn out the light and snuggle in under the covers, you just have to pause for a moment to know there is more to life than the physical events of the day. In the quiet of darkness, you *know*. If you review your day, you do not need some outside person or rule to decide the merits of your actions and thoughts. That small voice inside knows, and if you pause to listen for just a moment it tells you loud and clear.

Perhaps this is the most 'scary' thing of all. If there is some absolute version of wisdom, of Truth, of what is good and what is bad, and if this knowledge is within each one of us and we can have personal contact with it, then there is total accountability. This accountability need not be to any external arbitrator, for there is no one to trick, to lie to or to fool – no one but yourself.

Perhaps this is why some people instinctively avoid spiritual issues. It may be preferable to operate on the superficial, physical level of personality. While this type of existence is full of fear and can never lead to total well-being, many seem to be fooled into accepting it as the easiest option.

More and more people, however, are recognising the limitations of the materialist's world. Whereas, years ago, this search for spiritual reality was being paved by hippies and drop-outs who were turning their backs on the current society, now there is a new breed of seeker. In all walks of life, from humblest to most powerful, there is a growing urge to replace the meaning or purpose in life, and the recognition that this can only come with spirituality.

For now the urge is to express this spirituality in practical terms, by injecting a new-found enthusiasm and love into daily tasks and routines.

With it comes a new mood. From the conflict, which was a product of the fears that materialism engendered, springs a new sense of hope and cooperation.

Following on from the healing of individuals, we see healing of the planet. For it is part of the human condition that only when we feel ourselves to be in intimate union with something bigger than ourselves, to be a part of it and working in harmony with it, can we be truly happy. Once we do develop such a framework into which we fit, our life becomes comfortable and meaningful, a base line of inner well-being is assured.

In this lies the secret. We have this inner core which is often apart from our outer reality, our personality. When our life is preoccupied with mundane things, with the physical world and our personality, it remains ephemeral indeed. It is like living in the shadows. There is a constant sense of inner division. It is only when we recognise and commune with this inner reality that life attains the meaning we seek. When personality and soul are one, harmony is ours.

It should be clear that this search for a spiritual reality is an intensely personal one. It is not one that can be satisfied by the words of another. While there are many valuable signposts in the books and religions of the world, it is clear to modern man that only a direct and personal experience of things spiritual can satisfy an individual. It must come from within.

I am blessed to have an inkling of a sense of order in my life. I am in no way evangelical. I cannot see how I could be. When I stop to consider my writing in this area, I tremble a little. I consider myself to be a precocious student, full of enthusiasm for what I have experienced. I smile at my good fortune and, as I dare to share it, I trust to God that I do not make too many mistakes along the way.

What I have done is to develop a sense of order in my life. I have a personal concept of God, where I came from, what I am doing here and where I will go. In this framework I feel comfortable and it helps to make sense of what I experience. It has turned the trials of my life into opportunities rather than leaving them as problems, and nothing so far has been too big to face.

This is the point. We all do have a God – our God provides us with our basic belief system. So for some, their God is money or status in the material world. For some, God is a mythological character, remote and fearsome, who rules in an arbitrary and fierce way. For still others, it is the divine spark behind every manifestation of life. Whatever form your God takes, that is the thing which determines the range of your possibilities. It puts *order* into your life; it determines how you make basic decisions and it provides the ground rules for your existence. And, likewise, your God also provides you with limits. If money is your God, then you become limited to what you can buy and sell, own or give away. You are limited to a hundred dollars, a thousand, a million? This is a little God indeed!

My God is a Big God. Infinite. I see Him in all Creation. Whenever I need reassurance, I have only to walk out into a

paddock, get down on my knee, search in the grass, and wonder at
the myriads of minute life forms before me. What diversity, what
colour, shape and sound. What beauty. Then I look up, am struck
by the blaze of colours in the magnificent parrots of our forests,
and marvel afresh at joyous creation at work.

I have had glimpses of the depths of this creative force in those
precious moments of silent *meditation*. I see it radiated through
the natural, effervescent smiles of children. It touches my soul
when at home the sun sets in its resplendent glory, bathing the hills
in liquid, golden light and, as the darkness comes, the stars twinkle
forth to remind me of the vastness of our universe. Then I am
struck to the core at my individuality. To think I am conscious of
all this, this vast range of creativity at work, and yet *I* have been
created to express something a little different, to contribute
something to the whole! This causes me to wonder in awe, and to
respect myself and all those around me and to know that the love
that I have for myself is love for that Divine Spark within me, just
as it is within you.

I am drawn to the analogy of symphony music. As a novice in
the audience, we hear the sounds of a great symphony and can only
take in a brief span of each segment of music as it is played. Our
knowledge of what was before, and what is yet to come, is narrow
indeed. As we sit through the concert over and over, we come to
appreciate the total score. We note the recurring rhythms, and
while we can still appreciate the immediate section we are
listening to, we now see it as part of a cohesive whole. As we learn
more of music, we may begin to play our own instrument. At first
tentatively, and then with growing confidence, we can take our
part in the orchestra. Now we are creating music in our own right.
To the audience, we may only be one small part of a fabulous
symphony of sounds, but if we were not in tune the discord would
be obvious. So with all in tune, all playing their part, harmony is
the result.

Pause to consider something else. A symphony concert relies on
far more than the musicians. There are the stage hands, the ticket
sellers, the managers, the theatre cleaners, the audience, the taxi
drivers who transport the participants, and on and on. Each is
essential. The musicians may take the limelight, but what if the
lighting technicians were not present? What if the cleaners did not

perform? Each has his role to play, and each is dependent upon the other.

So, as I strive to sound my note in harmony, I recognise that the conductor in my life is this very important, very Big God. I have a relationship with this God that I value and work on. I commune with my God regularly and have come to know him as reliable – always there, always ready, always masterful. Whatever I need will always come to me. I know my life has a sense and structure, and I know that it is only when I get preoccupied with things of Personality and lose the Spiritual thread that I get problems.

Over the years I have been reassured further by the way our lives do run to a rhythm. I no longer believe in 'coincidences' as such, but continue to marvel at the Law of Synchronicity. So many things happen, so many people are met, just at the right time when they are needed most.

I see all in my life happening for good, not simply because I am a natural-born optimist, but because I have this sense of a Big God being at the core of my life. Because of the concept I have of my Big God, I feel confident that anything is possible. My God is infinite in size, limitless in scope.

As such, it is impossible to know this God in entirety. Like walking up to a vast sea, we can only comprehend a little of the whole, that little within our grasp. But there are some things I can appreciate.

First, I recognise a grand intelligence at work throughout the Universe as I know it. When you look at the vast realms of nature, from the minute to the massive, there seems to be intelligence at work. Again, this is a basic choice. Either you recognise that life is orderly, or you do not. The odds that all of life is merely the product of mathematical chance happenings must be huge indeed. I feel it takes more faith to ignore the probabilities, and be atheistic, than it does to delight in the presence of this unifying thread running through all creation.

So the first aspect that I can appreciate of my God is Intelligence. This universal consciousness gives life its basic structure and patterns. It is the grand consciousness of God that permeates all things, that provides the basic energy patterns which we interpret as matter. God projects Intelligence – His consciousness – like some master projectionist in a movie theatre.

Most of us are looking at the same screen, seeing the same movies. All of us have the capacity to affect the focus, the clarity of the picture. A rare few it seems, are able to project their own movies for others to see. It is consciousness that projects the pattern, while the mind interprets it. Conscious Intelligence is the first principle.

We then can see that there is a second basic force involved. For Intelligence to be functional, it must be just that; there must be action. Some people call it Force, or even Will, as it is Intelligence in Action. It is easy, however, to realise that this characteristic of Action is necessary. Imagine being just pure Intelligence. Imagine if you had been born into a black soundproof cupboard with no sensory input, nothing to do. What would you do? Something, of course! You would want to find a door, make a door, get out, do something. So Action is the second property.

Now, if you add pure Action to pure Intelligence, you can only produce one thing. Reflect on it. There is only one possibility: pure Love. So Love is the third quality that characterises God – it is pure Action based on pure Intelligence. These three things – Intelligence, Action, Love – are the Trinity that is expressed in virtually all major religions as being at the heart of their concept of God. So, in Christianity, there is God the Father, symbol of Divine Intelligence; God the Son – Jesus the Christ, symbol of Divine Love; and the Holy Spirit, symbol of God in action. In the Hindu religion there is Brahma – Intelligence, Krishna – Love, Shiva – Action.

From this, the world as we know it has been created by a pure Intelligence, acting through pure Love. The whole world, then, was created by Love and is sustained by Love. If this is so, why do we see so much disharmony?

Again we must look to the facts and observe a great deal of evidence of unloving action by man. How can this be so, if man and his world were created by pure Love? We must recognise another vital factor.

This one is easiest to understand when we consider the act of creation from our own viewpoint. Now, whether it is valid or not to assess an infinite God in our finite terms, is pure speculation, but the attempt for a rationale is worthwhile.

I used to keep Australian finches. These delightful little birds reflect an exquisite spectrum of God's creativity. In setting up an aviary, however, one almost reenacts the steps in Genesis. First one starts with the idea, the thought of creating an aviary and stocking it with birds. The planning over, a cage is built and then plants introduced, feeders and watering points added and filled. You create the best conditions you can imagine in which the birds will be happy. That done, you add the birds themselves.

Now, if you knew for sure that the birds would be happy, would thrive, would breed regularly and behave in a predictable manner, would you still approach the project with the same zest? Would you even bother? The real point of it, is to see how the occupants interact with their environment.

Satisfaction comes with adjusting the feed, the location of breeding boxes, and so on, until the birds do settle into this artificially created environment. Then, as they display their natural tendencies and you learn of their habits, watch them breed and share in their joy, your own joy is added to. The key is, the birds are free agents within the limits you have imposed. They are not going to react predictably, but they do respond to what is around them.

Was this God's motive? Who knows? It is fairly obvious, however, that – for whatever reason – man has free will. Born of pure spirit, man has been given his own consciousness and the free will to use it as he sees fit in a world that could be Heaven. Man has been given that unique combination of Spirit and Matter. Created in God's image, he has the potential to embody pure consciousness contained within a pure physical form. Jesus the Christ did just this. He was the representation of man fully realised, man's potential fully attained.

It would seem that mankind generally has been lured from the spiritual unity to explore the material world of the senses. By using his free will to make this choice, man has Fallen from the Heavenly God-consciousness to the fear-based worldliness we are so familiar with. With this Fall comes a separation from the Unity of God. With separation comes division; with division, opposites. So, as a natural consequence, follow the opposites of good and evil, pain and pleasure, joy and sorrow, health and disease. Even Man himself is divided, male and female again being a grand symbol of the opposites. In the union of conception however, this separation is overcome, unity is established – if only for an instant – and new life is created: all part of the mystery of life.

So what is the point? If these opposites are an inherent part of life, how do we avoid them? Should we avoid them? Obviously, if we could reunify with the whole, reunite with God, the opposites would no longer exist and we would know true harmony, true happiness. This is why anything that leads to wholeness, to balance, to harmony, is a healing agent and restores us to health. Man's destiny is conscious reunion with God – to become a happy musician in the symphony of Life.

Having such a view of my own spiritual reality, such a belief system, makes me feel personally accountable for my actions. It removes fear from my life and increases my level of well-being tremendously. It does, however, add the conscious conflict between spirit and personality. There is still some inner tension as I try to align the two. But I smile a whole lot more than I used to, and the smile comes from way down deep inside.

Would this philosophical scheme of mine work for another? This I cannot say. You must conduct your own inner search and, if your conclusions agree with mine, well and good. All I can say is that I have rediscovered something of great personal value. This inner conviction has carried me through what for many would be the ultimate challenge in life. I have had cancer, lost a leg, and come out smiling, feeling that everything was as it should be.

That, to me, is worthwhile.

My hope is that my message will encourage another to change the challenges in their life from problems into opportunities and to regain their true health.

CONCLUSION

So often we have met people who feel hopeless, as if there is nothing they can do to help themselves. Then, presented with all the very real possibilities we have been discussing, they soon find themselves wondering where to begin, how to fit it all in, what to do.

We expect individuals to vary, but in general the following would be a reasonable order of priorities for those looking to help themselves towards maximising their potentials.

For patients recently diagnosed and basically well

1   Answer the four basic question:
(a) Do I really want to get well again?

(b) Am I prepared to accept responsibility for my situation?

(c) Do I want to use toxic or non-toxic therapies?

(d) Which particular therapies shall I use?

Assess each therapy according to the principles:

(i) What are my expectations with no treatment?

(ii) What are the expectations for me if I have the proposed treatment?

(iii) Are there any side effects to the treatment and, if so, what might they be?

[Refer Chapter 1]

2   Medical treatment

If a specific therapy is suitable for you, and you decide to have it, commit yourself to it fully and work to minimise any potential side-effects and maximise its benefits.

3   Self-Help Techniques

(a) Meditation: This is the ideal first step because it deals with stress and makes it easier to act appropriately.

(i) If quality of life is your prime aim, begin with three sessions of ten to twenty minutes daily, and once it is working well, maintain two sessions of ten to twenty minutes daily.

(ii) If you want to gain maximum benefit from *meditation*, begin with three sessions daily of whatever period you feel comfortable with and build as rapidly as possible to three sessions of one hour each day.

[Refer Chapters 2 and 3.]

(b) Dietary considerations Once the *meditation* is becoming integrated into your day, consider your dietary choices:

(i) *Make no change*: The average Western diet is high in fat, protein, salt, sugar, alcohol and refined foods, low in fibre, and vitamin/mineral intakes may be inadequate. The 'average' person would do well, therefore, to consider change. Recognise that change in this vital area may be traumatic and stressful. Spend time to think it through, discuss it and be clear on your aims and choices. *Meditation* makes change easier. Seek professional guidance.

(ii) *The maintenance diet*: This is a good, sensible approach as it avoids known risk factors and concentrates on foods that we know to carry preventive factors or actively promote health. Essentially, it is low in fat, protein and alcohol, avoids salt, sugar and refined foods, and has a high fibre content. Its primary constituents are the fruits, vegetables and grains. For maximum benefit use the recommendations for the acute situation for the first two months. As your condition improves and you develop your own sensitivity as to what is best for you, gradually relax towards the basic maintenance recommendations. This then becomes a lifelong way of eating, with some latitude for special occasions if you feel the need.

(iii) *Individual Regeneration Program*: This is a more intense approach which is better suited to those who want to emphasise their dietary considerations. It relies on an initial mono-diet of three to ten days to give an element of fasting, detoxification, transition and regeneration. Then follows one, or preferably two months, of still quite intensive attention, followed by a gradual relaxation to the ongoing maintenance diet.

(iv) *Follow a specific, formal diet*: e.g. the Pritikin Program, Kelley's Diet, Anne Wigmore's approach, Contrere's diet (as in Edye Maye's book) or the Gerson Therapy. The last mentioned, particularly, is suited to a clinic situation and it is not recommended to be attempted at home without skilled guidance and the committed support of at least one permanent, full-time helper.

[Refer Chapters 6 and 7.]

(c) Positive Thinking: With *meditation* and Dietary Considerations, this completes the three basic ingredients of well-being. Recognise the basic need to be positive, affirm it, and use the techniques put forward as they seem appropriate for your situation. [See Chapter 5 for summary of ways of maintaining a positive attitude.] If you do feel depressed or negative, start by working on a creative activity. By actually doing something physical and positive, you will set the whole process in motion. Gardening is my favourite activity. Exercise also should get priority.

[Refer Chapter 4.]

(d) Spiritual Development: For most, this is another essential. Recognise that your endeavours in this area may be the most important of all.

(i) *Religion*: Follow your own preference here. Very few patients change their religion through an experience with disease, but many find their convictions strengthened.

(ii) *Reflection, Introspection, Contemplation*: Highly recommended as long as they are not associated with guilt or other negative emotions. Seek to understand your past, accept your present and work 'in the now' towards a happier, healthier tomorrow.

(iii) *Belief system*: Your belief system can limit your horizons or leave you free to soar above any situation with a smile on your face. Spend time reading, thinking, in contemplation, and in evolving your own theories. Open yourself to the possibilities.

(iv) *Spiritual Healing*: This may be catalysed by others, but often comes with personal experience. Learning to love that part of your inner self, the Divine within, is an integral part of loving God and your fellows. Once you can love yourself, you can recognize the Divine in others. Then you can see that they too are seeking to be free of limitations and to express the perfection of the Divine. So too you will realise that it is not enough to dwell in spirit. The body is the temple of the soul and you need to give it due consideration. *Healing is complete when harmony is found in body, mind and spirit.*

(e) Positive Emotions: Relationships frequently require as much healing as the physical body.

(i) *Make peace with as many as you can*. Use the visualisation technique of Release [See Chapter 5] once your *meditation* is working well.

(ii) *The immediate family may need all these principles just as much as you do*. Often it is the patient whose physical symptoms reflect a malaise involving one or several other closely associated people. Encourage your family to support you and to join you in as much of your program as possible, particularly the big three: *meditation*, diet and positive thinking. You may well find it easier than they do!

[Refer Chapter 10.]

(f) Pain Control: Another essential for all at some stage. Do the recommended pain control exercises and be aware of the other possibilities.

[See summary at the end of Chapter 6.]

(g) Consideration of Death and Dying: Another vitally important issue not to be evaded.

(i) Practicalities:

(1) Formulate your Will.

(2) Discuss your choices for terminal care, including:

● Preferred location, e.g. home, hospice or hospital.

● The extent to which life support systems should be used.

● Approach to use of drugs which may affect your degree of consciousness.

• Those you wish present – family, friends, medical staff, church people?

• Any special requirements: food, flowers, effects, music, etc.

(3) Plan for the future of those close to you:

• You may seek reassurance of their financial security.

• Express your preferences for their welfare, e.g. children's schooling, parenting, spouse remarrying, etc.

• Consider whether or not you want to leave tapes or written material for children to have at significant stages in their lives, e.g. for children at ages eighteen or twenty-one, at marriage, or on a first child's birth, etc.

(ii) Principles: Be brave enough to reflect and contemplate upon what you anticipate may happen. Look at your fears, if any. Actively seek the opportunity to discuss the whole area with a good listener and especially, if possible, with your closest relative. With the fears confronted and allayed, and with the benefit of regular *meditation* and contemplation, death can be genuinely seen as another very natural and positive part of life.

[Refer Chapter 11.]

(h) Healing: Be convinced that true healing lies within, and work towards your own wholeness with resulting health. However, healers who can act as catalysts in the process may be necessary and appropriate. Be aware of the possibilities and use your own judgement. We certainly *do not* recommend that anyone should jump in a plane and dash off to the Philippines, India or wherever. However, if you do seek healing help from an extraordinary source, find out as much as you can about it before you begin. Having made your choice, strive to be open to the best possible outcome and commit yourself to the requirements of the healing technique involved.

(i) Visualisation:
   • If you conscientiously apply yourself to *meditation* for three months and find it remains unsatisfactory because of persistent, acute, unavoidable thoughts interrupting your efforts to experience stillness, you may be better to take up this more active process of visualisation. You could use the gentle,

abstract methods such as the Revitalising Light Visualisation. If you choose to use a more aggressive image such as armies doing battle, make sure you seek qualified guidance. If you use either approach regularly, do them for ten to twenty minutes three times daily and keep at the back of your mind the desire to experience moments of stillness whenever possible. Seek to be as relaxed as you can be. Don't 'give up' on *meditation* too soon, as almost all people who persevere can do it, and it has special benefits.

[Refer Chapter 5.]

● Visualisation can be an 'optional extra' to *meditation* once the latter is going well. It does utilise the active, more forceful side of the mind, whereas *meditation* relies on the stillness. Again, gentle, abstract visualisation is safe and recommended; but you are strongly cautioned against active visualisation using images of conflict.

To repeat: A journey of a thousand miles begins with just one step.

For patients in a critical condition

The same basic approach applies. You may feel quality of life issues are more important than efforts to overcome your physical symptoms. In this case, both medical and self-help techniques may be counter-productive. Changes in diet may just cause anguish, whereas *meditation* always leads to peace of mind and remains the priority. Most people who use all the principles, find they apply to any life situation and so make for a good life – and a good death.

Faced with a crisis, your attitudes and beliefs assume paramount importance and peace of mind should be the basic aim. So do seek to avoid or resolve situations of conflict as the calm that follows is enduring. I would never abandon hope of conquering disease, as it is my firm belief that healing is possible in any situation. However, it is not completely cynical to say that while any disease is curable, some patients are not.

I am confident that the techniques we have discussed in the book work. *They only work if you apply them.* You can be helped greatly by individuals, groups, conducive environments, etc., but all these things we have talked about are blatantly self-help techniques.

You can greatly improve your situation. You can be confident of that. It is not reasonable, however, to expect that everyone will be freed of their physical symptoms. Some will need to look at dying, but success or failure is not marked by death. Success is marked by poise and equanimity. The greatest successes I have seen have been in people who have developed a strong, pro-life, I-choose-to-live-to-the-full stance, but at the same time have been able to accept what life had to offer in return, even if it is dying. However, a great many have become well, and virtually all who have applied themselves to the principles have felt a great deal of benefit. Any effort will be rewarded.

For those interested in prevention or in maximum health

Surprise! The same principles still apply. The degree to which you apply them depends on your priorities, beliefs and expectations.

As an ideal prevention programme which would lead to maximum health, I would recommend confidently:

(a) *Meditation*: Ten to twenty minutes twice daily.

(b) *Diet*: Basic Maintenance diet.

(c) *Positive Thinking*: Keep developing this, using the techniques already summarised.

(d) *Make time* – yes, *make* time – to dwell on and implement the recommendations for spiritual development, positive emotions, pain control, considerations of death and dying, and healing. Visualisation may find a place in your programme.

I am confident that these basic, self-help principles and techniques will find application in virtually all conditions. They may be applied to other disease states besides those of cancer or merely used as aids to maximise health.

Make total health your goal. Make that elusive, ephemeral, wonderful, joyous state of harmony in body, mind and soul your life ambition. Seek to develop your potentials to the full.

Be patient, yet persevere for the goal is real and within reach. Be gentle with yourself. Most have ups and downs along the way. Remember, it is your belief system which validates your actions. If your actions are not in line with your belief system, you are almost certain to produce disease. You may have pondered on boozing, smoking and shuffling-old-George who probably thinks that his life is okay and so has no inner conflict. By doing so he accepts sub-standard health. But while he may have no obvious physical symptoms of disease, his version of health is a pale image of his potential.

Once you have a glimpse of *your* true potential and realise that we are all destined for an ultimate state of perfection, you will feel the urge to achieve it. Accept that it takes time. Making a start and being on the path to true health in body, mind and spirit will transform your life and bring you peace. Life *was* meant to be good.

Happiness should be found along the way, not just at the end of the path.

Appendix A

DIETARY ANALYSIS

To examine the nutrient content of the diets we use, we had them analysed by Dietary Analysis (Aust.) at 595 Whitehorse Road, Mitcham, Victoria. They use a computer model based on the Australian Food Exchange Tables. Where no Australian values are available, they use British tables. They then base comparisons on the Recommended Daily Allowances set down for nutrients by the Australian Department of Health. There are some problems. We found that there were some things we normally use in our diet for which the computer did not have values, also the bread figures used are based on salted breads which, therefore, dramatically raise their sodium levels. But, overall, this is the best analysis that we know about. This service of Dietary Analysis is available to the public and is reasonably priced at under $20, so if you wish to analyse the content of your own diet, this service is well worth considering.

We analysed samples of our maintenance diet as being used by: (1) a 50 kg female with light activity; (2) the same diet and six juices; (3) the Gerson diet as applied to a 70 kg male with light activity. The results are summarised and show a supplement of Vitamins E, B_{12} and Zinc may be useful. Perhaps this is another indication for a multi-vitamin formula which assures an adequate supply of all these vital nutrients.

The maintenance diet came out low in energy. We certainly see people lose excess weight in this diet, but our experience is that it stabilises at a lean, fit level. If lack of energy was experienced or weight loss continued, it could be easily rectified by eating more carbohydrates.

It should be noted that the figures given are the result of examining a *three day* sample diet.

212 *You can conquer cancer*

LEGEND

PROT	= Protein
CHO	= Carbohydrate (Sugars & Starch)
ENGY	= Energy
Ca	= Calcium
I'	= Phosphorus
Fe	= Iron
Na	= Sodium (Constituent of ordinary salt)
K	= Potassium
B-CRT	= Beta Carotene (orange plant pigment)
RETIN	= Retinol (Vitamin A)
B_1	= Vitamin B_1 (Thiamine)
B_2	= Vitamin B_2 (Riboflavin)
NIACIN	= Vitamin B_3 (Niacin)
VIT-C	= Vitamin C
VIT-E	= Vitamin E
B_6	= Vitamin B_6 (Pyridoxine)
B_{12}	= Vitamin B_{12}
Zn	= Zinc
FIBRE	= Dietary Fibre
CHOL	= Cholesterol
FOLIC	= Folic Acid
Mg	= Magnesium
g	= gram weight
mg	= milligram weight
mcg	= microgram weight
kJ	= kilojoules
4.2 kJ	= 1 Calorie
RDA	= Recommended Daily Allowance

*   Includes RETINOL produced in the body from B-CAROTENE.

**   Includes NIACIN produced in the body from TRYPTOPHAN.

*** RDA's have not been set for these nutrients. However, dietary goals do exist for some of them.

Maintenance Diet – 50 kg Female

		Supplied by Diet	Recommended (RDA)	% of RDA (Diet/RDA *100)
WATER	gm	1535.88	***	
PROT	gm	62.02	55.11	113
FAT	gm	52.36	***	
CHO	gm	325.71	***	
ENGY	kJ	8080.74	9184.80	88
ENGY	Cal	1930.42	2194.17	
Ca	mg	870.64	400.00	218
P	mg	1298.73	**	
Fe	mg	20.44	12.00	170
Na	mg	2418.24	***	
K	mg	5493.97	***	
B-CRT	mcg	21330.11	***	
RETIN	mcg	112.83		
RETIN*	mcg	3667.85	750.00	489
B_1	mcg	1577.20	918.48	172
B_2	mcg	1661.87	1102.18	151
NIACIN	mg	14.97		
NIACIN**	mg	24.90	14.70	169
VIT-C	mg	274.39	30.00	915
VIT-E	mg	11.33	12.00	94
VIT-B_6	mcg	2837.73	2000.00	142
VIT-B_{12}	mcg	.80	2.00	40
Zn	mg	10.51	15.00	70
FIBRE	gm	62.88	20.00	314
CHOL	mg	123.00	300.00	41
FOLIC	mcg	627.67	200.00	314
Mg	mg	629.50	300.00	210

% of Total Energy in the diet provided by:

1. PROTEIN = 12.3 (Recommended = 10 to 12%)
2. FAT = 23.3 (Recommended = 30 to 35%)
3. CHO = 64.4 (Recommended = 55 to 60%)

Energy (DIET) = 8081 kJ (1930 Cals)
Energy (RDA) = 9185 kJ (2194 Cals)

Difference (DIET — RDA):
= 1104 kJ (264 Cals)

If the diet record is accurate and is typical of the patient's diet for the rest of the week, then the above energy difference would result in the patient LOSING .2 kg (.5 lbs) per week.

Maintenance and Juices – 50 kg Female

		Supplied by Diet	Recommended (RDA)	% of RDA (Diet/RDA *100)
WATER	gm	2795.93	***	
PROT	gm	75.08	55.11	136
FAT	gm	54.98	***	
CHO	gm	499.33	***	
ENGY	kJ	11001.48	9184.80	120
ENGY	Cal	2628.16	2194.17	
Ca	mg	1387.75	400.00	347
P	mg	1745.93	***	
Fe	mg	30.94	12.00	258
Na	mg	3043.75	***	
K	mg	9475.91	***	
B-CRT	mcg	75950.76	***	
RETIN	mcg	252.83		
RETIN*	mcg	12911.29	750.00	1722
B$_1$	mcg	2505.44	1100.15	228
B$_2$	mcg	2467.31	1320.18	187
NIACIN	mg	21.97		
NIACIN**	mg	33.99	17.60	193
VIT-C	mg	561.56	30.00	1872
VIT-E	mg	12.63	12.00	105
VIT-B$_6$	mcg	3226.73	2000.00	161
VIT-B$_{12}$	mcg	.80	2.00	40
Zn	mg	11.67	15.00	78
FIBRE	gm	69.18	20.00	346
CHOL	mg	123.00	300.00	41
FOLIC	mcg	915.67	200.00	458
Mg	mg	792.00	300.00	264

% of Total Energy in the diet provided by:

1. PROTEIN = 10.8 (Recommended = 10 to 12%)
2. FAT   = 17.7 (Recommended = 30 to 35%)
3. CHO   = 71.5 (Recommended = 55 to 60%)

Energy (DIET) = 11001 kJ (2628 Cals)
Energy (RDA) = 9185 kJ (2194 Cals)

Difference (DIET — RDA):
            = 1817 kJ   (434 Cals)

If the diet record is accurate and is typical of the patient's diet for the rest of the week, then the above energy difference would result in the patient GAINING .4 kg (.9 lbs) per week.

Gerson Diet – 70 kg Male

		Supplied by Diet	Recommended (RDA)	% of RDA (Diet/RDA *100)
WATER	gm	4121.97	***	
PROT	gm	164.90	69.90	236
FAT	gm	95.00	***	
CHO	gm	642.35	***	
ENGY	kJ	16312.36	11650.00	140
ENGY	Cal	3896.88	2783.09	
Ca	mg	1659.12	400.00	415
P	mg	3743.34	***	
Fe	mg	86.09	10.00	861
Na	mg	4091.26	***	
K	mg	15108.84	***	
B-CRT	mcg	99999 Plus	***	
RETIN	mcg	41914.20		
RETIN*	mcg	69373.41	750.00	9250
B_1	mcg	4852.52	1631.24	297
B_2	mcg	17875.20	1957.48	913
NIACIN	mg	105.20		
NIACIN**	mg	131.58	26.10	504
VIT-C	mg	927.28	30.00	3091
VIT-E	mg	13.20	15.00	88
VIT-B_6	mcg	6073.00	2000.00	304
VIT-B_{12}	mcg	500.00	2.00	9999 Plus
Zn	mg	50.27	15.00	335
FIBRE	gm	62.14	20.00	311
CHOL	mg	1850.00	300.00	617
FOLIC	mcg	2268.37	200.00	1134
Mg	mg	969.68	350.00	277

% of Total Energy in the diet provided by:

1. PROTEIN = 16.2 (Recommended = 10 to 12%)
2. FAT = 20.9 (Recommended = 30 to 35%)
3. CHO = 62.9 (Recommended = 55 to 60%)

Energy (DIET) = 16312 kJ (3897 Cals)
Energy (RDA) = 11650 kJ (2783 Cals)

Difference (DIET — RDA):
= 4662 kJ (1114 Cals)

If the diet record is accurate and is typical of the patient's diet for the rest of the week, then the above energy difference would result in the patient GAINING 1.0 kg (2.2 lbs) per week.

Appendix B

REJUVELAC

Take one cup of organically grown wheat:

1 Wash wheat, rinsing thoroughly until water is clear.
2 Soak one volume wheat in three volumes water for forty-eight hours.
3 Pour off liquid and keep – this is the first Rejuvelac batch.
4 Using the same seed, add another three volumes of water and soak for only twenty-four hours.
5 Pour off liquid – this is the second batch.
6 Repeat steps four and five once more, then discard seed and begin again at step 1.

Batches of Rejuvelac may be stored in the refrigerator for several days. It should have a pleasant odour and a lemon-like flavour. If it is offensive it should be discarded. It can be used as a drink in lieu of water or added to cooking.

Appendix C

CAFFEINE ENEMAS

1   Use only fresh ground coffee beans.

2   Add 2 tablespoons to 1 pint of water, bring to the boil and simmer for ten minutes.

3   Cool to body temperature, and filter into enema bag. Use a gravity fed type of bag.

4   Go to the toilet first if necessary. When first using enemas you may benefit from a wash out enema of plain water to evacuate the bowel before the caffeine enema is administered, but this is not necessary routinely.

5   If insecure, lie on a plastic sheet. Most people can retain an enema quite easily, especially if they relax.

6   Lie on your right side with your legs tucked up a little. Consciously **relax**.

7   Insert the enema tube's lubricated nozzle through the anus and gently allow the liquid to flow in.

8   Switch off the flow and remove the nozzle.

9   **Relax** for ten to fifteen minutes while retaining the enema. Reading is a good distraction if you need it.

10   Go to the toilet and evacuate the bowel.

11   Be sure to wash your enema equipment thoroughly after every use.

Appendix D

DIETARY REGIME FOR SMALL ANIMALS WITH CANCER

This article was first published in the 'Control and Therapy' articles of the Post Graduate Committee in Veterinary Science Publication, University of Sydney and has since been slightly revised.

Does this sound familiar? 'Your dog has cancer, there is nothing we can do. Shall we euthanase him now or later?'

This is a précis of an often repeated if more gently expressed diagnosis and sentence. It leaves the animal and owner without professional support, and likely to prematurely terminate a loved pet's life or to seek help from unqualified alternative sources. It leaves the practitioner missing out on an opportunity to follow through a stimulating and helpful exercise in disease management.

Having been through it myself with osteogenic sarcoma and having felt the benefits that dietary considerations offer, I have developed a dietary regime that I am confident offers help to animals with cancer. I present it on the basis of clinical experimentation with the knowledge that it does improve the quality of the animal's life. It has not cured anything as yet, although it has been instrumental in several remissions. I do feel, however, that it has prolonged life in many cases and am certain it has made the most of a difficult situation. It has also eased many people's minds when they want to do something constructive instead of just watching their animals die. Many owners comment on how fit and active their animals are despite the presence of tumours. Also, when the diet is followed, it is frequently noted that the animal's demise, when it comes, is rapid. Rather than a drawn out, steady deterioration frequently associated with cancer, the animal remains well, often fitter than usual, until there is a sudden collapse. Then, if a decision regarding euthanasia is required, it is usually easily made.

Overall, the diet has many positive attributes. The principles are to detoxify the body, correct mineral imbalances, restore the digestion and to develop and maintain a positive attitude. I have included Vitamin C as I believe there is plenty of good evidence to do so. Also included is the optional use of Laevamisole in the hope that it will boost the immune system. It seems to me to be helpful, although in light of recent articles I leave it as an option.

The diet recognises that we are dealing with carnivores, but that protein intake should be restricted. Gerson believed that cancer patients have an excess of salt and subsequent lack of potassium and iodine in an ultra-cellular level. Hence no salt and supplements of potassium and iodine.

Here it is:
Basic Components:
Meat 40% by volume (stewing steak type).

Vegetables 40% volume – concentrate on yellow ones, e.g. pumpkin, carrot, and green ones, cooked as little as possible.

Brown rice 20% volume – well cooked.

Presented as a stew; meat and vegetables cooked as little as acceptance dictates, e.g. generally well cooked to begin with and as palate adapts cook less – especially carrot and greens good if given raw – just grate finely.

Fed to appetite demands, once daily.

Fast one day per week.

Additives: for 15 kgm dog.
(a) 1 teaspoon cold pressed vegetable oil – sunflower or maize – added after cooking.
(b) ¼ teaspoon kelp powder or granules – pre-soaked or cooked with rice.
(c) 1 tablespoon brewer's yeast – not a bitter variety – add to stew.
(d) 3 drops Lugol's iodine – add to stew or drinking water.
(e) 200 mgm Potassium Orotate Bioglan – crumble onto stew.
(f) 1 Acidol Pepsin tablet Winthrop Laboratories – give by mouth.

(g) 2 Viokase tablets A. H. Robins – give by mouth.

(h) ½ Oroxine 100 mcgm tablet Wellcome Aust. – give by mouth.

(i) ½ teaspoon Sodium ascorbate powder – direct from CSR Chemicals in 5 kgm lots, or available in small packs from health food shops or chemists – sprinkle onto stew – generally accepted. If not I use Vita Glow Enteric coated 500 mg tablets and give 4 tablets.

Dogs generally accept the diet readily, cats more reluctantly. Its implementation requires a lot of owner participation and tends to lead to the vet becoming intimately involved in the whole procedure. It can be used as an adjunct in the treatment of any chronic degenerative disease.

I would welcome feedback.

REFERENCES

1   Doll, R. and Peto, R., *Causes of Cancer*, 1981, Oxford University Press, New York.

2   Meares, A., *Relief Without Drugs*, 1968, Souvenir Press, U.K.

3   Simonton, O. C., and Matthew, S., *Getting Well Again*, 1978, Bantam, New York.

4   Ramacharaka, Y., *Raja Yoga*, 1960, Lowe and Brydone (and Fowler), U.K.

5   Cousins, N., *Anatomy of an Illness*, 1979, Bantam, New York.

6   Ibid.

7   Doll and Peto, op cit.

8   Gerson, M., *A Cancer Therapy; Results of Fifty Cases*, 1958, Totality Books, California, U.S.A.

9   Ibid.

10 Kidman, B. O., *A Gentle Way With Cancer*, 1983, Century, London.

11 Pauling, L., and Cameron, E., *Cancer and Vitamin C*, 1979, Linus Pauling Institute of Science and Medicine, New York.

12 Minchin, M., *Food For Thought*, 1982, Alma Productions, St Arnaud, Australia.

13 Brand, J., *The Grape Cure*, Provoker Press, Canada.

14 Doll and Peto, op cit.

15 Le Shan, L., *You Can Fight For Your Life*, 1973, Turnstone Books, U.K.

16 Simonton and Matthews, of cit

17 Ibid.

18 Kubler-Ross, E., *On Death and Dying*, 1969, Macmillan, New York.

19 Moody, R., *Life After Life*, 1979, Bantam, New York.

20 Tompkins, P., and Bird, C., *The Secret Life of Plants*, Penguin, Australia.

FURTHER READING

'Note to *References and Further Reading:* This book is the product of stillness of mind. While personal experience, the experience of others and reading have made their contributions, its essence has been distilled in silence. It is a product or experiencing wholeness through meditation, and a product of experiencing life as order, not disorder. I regard this as a direct perception and so have used little documentation throughout the book. I regard the book as a personal guide to total health, and back its words by stating that they have worked for me, and for others. With this said, I acknowledge many books as having been very useful and I offer this list of books for highly recommended further reading, hoping that they will serve as introductions to a deeper exploration of their topics.

Meditation and Relaxation:

Meares, A., *Relief Without Drugs*, 1968, Souvenir Press and Fontana, Great Britain.

— *The Wealth Within*, 1978, Hill of Content, Melbourne.

Yoga:

Ramacharaka, Y., *Raja Yoga*, 1960, Lowe and Brydone, London.

Fowler, *Science of Breath*, 1904, Yogi Publishing Society, Chicago.

Dietary Considerations: Basic Information:

Urs Koch, M., *Laugh With Health*, 1981, Renaissance and New Age Creations, Metung, Australia.

Pritikin, N.,   *Pritikin's Diet and Exercise Program*, Grosset & Dunlop, Bantam, New York.

Phillips, D. A.,   *From Soil to Psyche*, 1977, Woodbridge Press, California.

Horne, R.,   *The New Health Revolution*, 1983, Happy Landings Publishing, Australia.

Kloss, J.,   *The Back to Eden Cookbook*, 1974, Woodbridge Press, California.

Hall, D.   *The Dorothy Hall Herb Tea Book*, 1980, Pythagorean Press, Sydney, Australia.

Minchin, M.,   *Food for Thought*, 1982, Alma Productions, St Arnaud, Australia.

Pauling, L., and Cameron, E.,   *Cancer and Vitamin C*, 1979, Linus Pauling Institute of Science and Medicine, New York.

Specialised Regimes:
Gerson, M.,   *A Cancer Therapy – Results of 50 Cases*, 1958, Totality Books, California.

Kidman, B.,   *A Gentle Way With Cancer*, 1983, Century, London.

Michio, Kushi,   *Cancer and Heart Disease*, 1982, Japan Publications, Tokyo.

Finkel, M.,   *Fresh Hope in Cancer*, 1978, Health Science Press, Bradford, England.

Brandt, J.,   *The Grape Cure*, Provoker Press, Ontario, Canada.

Wicks, J.,   *Guide to Exercise*, 1983, National Heart Foundation of Australia, Melbourne.

Causes of Cancer:
Doll, R., and Peto, R.,   *Causes Of Cancer*, 1981, Oxford University Press, New York.

Le Shan, L.,   *You Can Fight For Your Life*, 1978, Jove Publishing, U.S.A.

Simonton, O. C., and Matthews, S.,   *Getting Well Again*, 1978, Bantam, New York.

| Winter, R., | *Cancer Causing Agents*, 1979, Crown, New York. |
| Airola, P., | *Cancer: The Total Approach*, 1972, Health Plus, Arizona. |

Death and Dying:

Kubler-Ross, E.,	*On Death and Dying*, 1969, Macmillan, New York.
Moody, R.,	*Life After Life*, 1979, Bantam, New York.
Levine, S.,	*Who Dies?* 1982, Anchor Books, New York.

Healing Principles:

Cousins, N.,	*Anatomy Of An Illness*, 1979, Norton Publishing Co., Bantam, New York.
Jampolsky, G. G.,	*Love Is Letting Go Of Fear*, 1979, Celestial Arts, California.
Shinn, F. S.,	*The Game of Life and How to Play It*, 1925, Lowe & Brydone, Fowler & Co., Great Britain.
Simonton, O. C., and Matthews, S.,	*Getting Well Again*, 1978, Bantam, New York.

Introductions to Natural Methods and Techniques:

Blackie, M. G.,	*The Challenge of Homeopathy*, 1976, Unwin Paperbacks, London, and MacDonald & Jane as *The Patient, Not The Cure*.
Chancellor, P. M.,	*Handbook of the Bach Flower Remedies*, 1971, C. W. Daniel Co. Limited, London.
Hall, D.,	*Iridology*, 1980, Thomas Nelson, Australian.
Ramacharaka, Y.,	*The Science of Psychic Healing*, 1960, Fowler, London.

Gardening:

| Dean, E., | *Esther Dean's Gardening Book*, 1977, Harper & Row, Australia. |

Fukuoka, M., *The One Straw Revolution*, Rodale Press, U.K. First published as *Shizen Noho Wara Ippon No Kakumei* by Hakujusha Co. Ltd., Tokyo, Japan.

Mollison, B., and Holmgren, D., *Permaculture One*, 1978, Corgi, Melbourne.

Mollison, B., Permaculture Two, 1979, Tagari Books, Australia.

Inspiration:

Bach, R., *Illusions – The Adventures of a Reluctant Messiah*, 1977, William Heinemann, Pan, Great Britain.

Bancroft, A., *Twentieth Century Mystics and Sages*, 1976, Henry Regnery Co., Chicago.

Capra, F., *The Tao of Physics*, 1976, Shambhala, Colorado, Bantam, New York.

Griffiths, B., *Return to the Centre*, 1976, Collins, Fount Paperbacks, Isle of Man, British Isles.

Hawken, P., *The Magic of Findhorn*, 1975, Harper & Row, Fontana, U.S.A.

Johnson, R. C., *The Imprisoned Splendour*, 1953, Harper & Row, New York, Quest Printing, U.S.A.

Meares, A., *Cancer Another Way*, 1977, Hill of Content, Melbourne.

— *From the Quiet Place*, 1976, Hill of Content, Melbourne.

— *Strange Places – Simple Truths*, 1969, Souvenir Press and Fontana, Great Britain.

— *Thoughts*, 1980, Hill of Content, Melbourne.

Sandweiss, S. H., *Sai Baba – The Holy Man And The Psychiatrist*, 1975, Birth Day Publishing Co., California.

Tompkins, P., and Bird, C., *The Secret Life of Plants*, 1974, Penguin, Australia.

The following article on Ian Gawler appeared in The Medical Journal of Australia 1978 2:433

The patient, aged 25, underwent a mid-thigh amputation for osteogenic sarcoma 11 months before he first saw me 2½ years ago. He had visible bony lumps of about 2 cm in diameter growing from the ribs, sternum and the crest of the ilium, and was coughing up small quantities of blood in which, he said, he could feel small spicules of bone. There were gross opacities in the X-ray films of his lungs. The patient had been told by a specialist that he had only two or three weeks to live, but in virtue of his profession he was already well aware of the pathology and prognosis of his condition. Now 2½ years later, he has moved to another State to resume his former occupation.

This young man has shown an extraordinary will to live and has sought help from all the alternatives to orthodox medicine which were available to him. These have included acupuncture, massage, several sessions with Philippine faith healers, laying on of hands and yoga in an Indian ashram. He had short sessions of radiation therapy, and chemotherapy, but declined to continue treatment. He has also persisted with the dietary and enema treatment prescribed by Max Gerson, the German, physician, who gained some notoriety for this type of treatment in America in the 1940s. However, in addition to all these measures to gain relief, the patient has consistently maintained a rigorous discipline of intensive meditation as described previously. He has in fact, consistently meditated from one to three hours daily.

Two other factors seem to be important. He has had extraordinary help and support from his girl friend, who more recently became his wife. She is extremely sensitive to his feelings and needs, and has spent hours in aiding his meditation and healing with massage and laying on of hands.

The other important factor would seem to be the patient's own state of mind. He has developed a degree of calm about him which I have rarely observed in anyone, even in oriental mystics with whom I have had some considerable experience. When asked to what he attributes the regression of metastases, he answers in some such terms as: "I really think it as our life, the way we experience our life". In other words, it would seem that the patient has let the effects of the intense and prolonged meditation enter into his whole experience of life. His extraordinarily low level of anxiety is obvious to the most casual observer. It is suggested that this has enhanced the activity of his immune system by reducing his level of cortisone.

Ainslie Meares, M.D.D.P.M.

[Since this report was written the patient has been declared free of active neoplastic disease — A.M.]

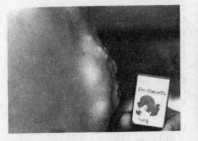
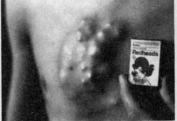

Photographs of the patient's chest taken on July 7, 1977.

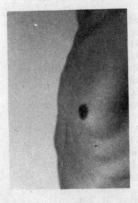
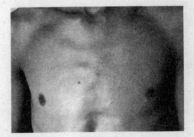

Recent photographs of the patient's chest.

INDEX

232 *You Can Conquer Cancer*

Index by John E. Simkin, Registered Indexer, Australian Society of Indexers.